HOW I
GAVE UP MY
LOW-FAT DIET
AND # LOST
40 POUNDS...
AND # HOW
YOU CAN TOO!

HOW I GAVE UP MY LOW-FAT DIET AND LOST 40 POUNDS... AND HOW YOU CAN TOO!

The Ultimate Guide to Low-Carbohydrate Dieting

DANA CARPENDER

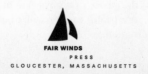

FAIR WINDS
PRESS
GLOUCESTER, MASSACHUSETTS

Text ©2003 by Dana Carpender

Second edition published in 2003 by
Fair Winds Press
33 Commercial Street
Gloucester, Massachusetts 01930-5089

First edition published in the U.S.A. in 1999 by
Hold the Toast Press
P.O. Box 6581
Bloomington, IN 47407

Library of Congress Cataloging-in-Publication Data available

Second Edition
10 9 8 7 6 5 4 3 2 1

ISBN 1-59233-040-1

Cover design by Stefan Killen design
Design by Leslie Haimes

Printed and bound in Canada

The information in this book is for educational purposes only.
It is not intended to replace the advice of a physician or medical practitioner. Please see your health care provider before
beginning any new health program.

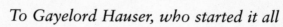

To Gayelord Hauser, who started it all

Contents

Foreword

I don't think there's any such thing as a coincidence. It's my belief that we get what we need when we need it and sometimes we just get what we deserve. I must have done something right because Dana Carpender came into my life and nothing has been the same since.

I must admit, I don't like to diet, especially if I have to measure, starve, eat things I don't like, or exercise. (I always say "Every time I feel like exercising, I lay down until the urge passes.") This has been the first diet I have actually enjoyed. I didn't—and still don't—measure, starve, eat things I don't like, or, most importantly to me, exercise. One more point before I tell what happened to me: It doesn't feel like dieting because after all those years of living on that dangerous low-fat "safe" diet, I always feel like I'm cheating, not dieting!

It was *Guiding Light* that did it, that infamous afternoon soap opera. I met Dana on a discussion list for *Guiding Light* on the Internet. We were all arguing about foods that are good and bad for us, meat in particular. I was saying how I tried to never eat meat because it was so dangerous healthwise, and everyone agreed except this maverick named Dana. This crazy woman was trying to convince me to eat not only meat, but lots of eggs!

I have serious kidney disease. No protein allowed! Imagine my outrage after eight years of starving and suffering on a low-fat diet. I had worked all those years on a low-fat diet to get my cholesterol down to 413 (from 990), my triglycerides to almost 1300 (from almost 1500), my blood pressure to 140/110, my creatinine (kidney function, normal at about 1) to 5, my blood urea nitrogen to 81, and my HDL to 24. What a reward for eight years of low-fat misery. I was a stroke waiting to happen until Dana completely changed my life.

To prove her wrong (My mission in life: To prove any woman wrong), I told her I would go on this silly diet and as soon as I gained five pounds, I would be done with it. I needed an excuse to eat all that wonderful, decadent stuff. Also, considering that my kidney disease causes outrageous cholesterol and triglyceride readings for which, my doctor informed me, there was nothing I could do—I was sure this craziness couldn't help. Dana gave me a long list of items to eat, and proper vitamins as well, carefully working around the limitations of my disease.

As you recall, I don't measure what I eat, so I just ate from the list she provided me. I did not ask my doctor about this diet, which I know is a no-no, but he never would have condoned such a thing. My hindsight and blood work tell me I made the right decision. I started to eat all the things my doctor had told me NOT to eat. I really wasn't nervous because I was certain I would gain the five pounds in a day or two, and the whole fiasco would be over. NOT!

I lost a pound a day for twenty days. Dana labeled me "carbohydrate intolerant." (I thought I was intolerant only of people.) I had gotten down to 212 pounds from 250 on low fat over the eight years, but I was stuck at that 212 and couldn't shake it no matter how many fruits and veggies I crammed down. I was ecstatic about the weight loss, getting down to 192 on Dana's method. However, I was quite worried about my upcoming blood work in a couple of days. Surely twenty days on a "fad diet" like this—eating three eggs a day, lots of meat, veggies, and piles of real butter and olive oil—couldn't alter my blood work that drastically, at least not for the better. NOT (again)!

Here are my results after this short period of time: My cholesterol was down almost 100 points to 337; my triglycerides were down more than 50 percent to 606; my blood pressure was normal for the first time since I was eighteen years old; my creatinine, which was up to 6.5 at one time and had remained steady at a horrible 5 for three years, had actually gone down to an astonishing 4.4; my BUN was slightly up at 92; and my HDL was reaching almost normal range at 33. All of these figures got even better in the three months following, but this shows how fast your body changes when it receives the proper foods.

It's been ten months since Dana saved me. (Am I an evangelist?) I've cheated some, eating that damn cancerous sugar on occasion, but holding my own pretty well. I love this way of eating because it's so easy to keep my weight stable. My cholesterol, considering my kidney disease and how it affects my blood work, is quite good in the 300 area. My triglycerides will rise a little if I cheat by eating sugar, but it's good to know they drop again quickly when I behave. They're still high, but good considering my kidney disease. My BUN is at its lowest in eight years at 65. My blood pressure is normal to *low*. My HDL is now in the normal range at 41. All this happened after thirty-something years of high blood pressure, two mild strokes by the age of forty-four, and hating diets, especially low fat. Go figure.

I used to take three Percocets and a sleeping pill every night just to get to sleep. My legs are really bad from the kidney disease, and I can't get to sleep. Now I'm down to two Percocets and half a sleeping pill, hoping to get down to one Percocet eventually. Between Dana's diet and my newfound magnet therapy, my leg pain is virtually gone. I stopped taking my blood pressure pill (again without telling my doctor) after one month on this diet, and also discontinued my strongest diuretic, continuing with just the weaker one. I have always abhorred drugs, and I'm now taking fewer drugs than I ever have since the onset of my kidney disease in 1990.

I've thanked Dana a thousand times since we met on the Internet. Someday I'll thank her in person with a big hug instead of only a cyberhug. Most of the folks on our *Guiding Light* discussion list still think we're fanatics or lunatics eating all of this type of food. I have fond memories of thinking the same thing about Dana a year ago. Everyone I know who has done this diet correctly has had great success, even more for health reasons than weight loss. I read a book many years ago that stated that the largest percentage of illness is actually caused by what we eat, and now I believe it.

Rob Douvres
Cape Coral, Florida

AUTHOR'S NOTE: *Although I support Rob's right to take his own risks and make his own judgments regarding his health, I can't endorse the idea of folks with health problems not consulting their doctors before making major changes in their health regimen. Please keep in mind that Rob did get blood work done regularly, to alert him to any potential problems.*

Introduction

Hi. My name is Dana Carpender. I'd like to tell you about a strange, unanticipated experience I had eight years ago now—how I gave up my low-fat diet and lost forty pounds. But first, I'd like to share two thoughts:

"If you always do what you've always done, you will always get what you have always got."

Definition of insanity: Doing the same thing over and over, while hoping for different results.

Before I tell you my story, here's a little quiz.

TRUE OR FALSE:

_____ I have been pretty faithful about cutting fat out of my diet and increasing complex carbohydrates.

_____ I have had a struggle to lose weight on a low-fat diet, or to maintain my weight loss.

_____ I think I am addicted to food.

_____ I work out mostly because if I didn't, I'd be *gaining* weight.

_____ I am hungry all the time and don't know why.

_____ I am frequently tired and cranky and don't know why.

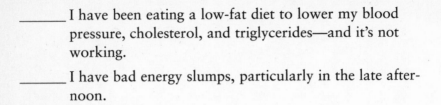

_____ I have been eating a low-fat diet to lower my blood pressure, cholesterol, and triglycerides—and it's not working.

_____ I have bad energy slumps, particularly in the late afternoon.

If you answered "true" to one or more of these questions, you're not alone! When I've asked these questions of groups of dieters, almost every hand in the room goes up!

If you've been wondering what the heck is wrong with you, that your healthy weight-loss diet just doesn't make you slim and healthy, or why you're hungry *all the time*, no matter how much you eat, take heart. IT'S NOT YOU! It's the diet. There is a very large group of people for whom a low-fat, high–complex carbohydrate diet is exactly the WRONG approach to weight loss and health. And the more of those questions you answered yes to, the more likely it is that you are one of those people. That's the good news. Here's the better news: I can teach you the *right* diet for people like us. I can teach you how to eat so that you lose weight. You'll eat real food, not strange, manufactured low-fat stuff, or packaged diet club meals. You'll be able to eat in restaurants and fast-food places. You'll have more energy than you ever dreamed possible. Your moods will improve till you wonder where all that cheerfulness is coming from! And maybe best of all, you won't be hungry all the time. *In fact, you'll be so un-hungry, you'll be amazed!*

Sound good? It's better than just good. It's fantastic, incredible, unbelievable—and TRUE! I've been living this way for eight years now. Not only have I lost forty pounds and kept it off, but I've watched my friends and family have incredible success with this way of eating. And through the magic of the Internet, I've found hundreds more folks for whom these dietary principles have made the difference between obesity and fatigue and vibrant, energetic trimness!

So if you're ready to look and feel better than you ever have before, turn the page and read on.

CHAPTER ONE

Here's What Happened to Me

In February 1995, I was trying to lose weight for my wedding. Despite active work (I'm a massage therapist by trade) and a low-fat, high–complex carbohydrate diet, I had gotten up to 175 pounds at 5′2″. I signed up at the local municipal fitness center and started doing four to five step aerobics classes a week. I cut back even further on my fat, and substituted grains for meat a lot. (You know the drill—cutting up one low-fat turkey smoked sausage in a huge casserole of potatoes, with low-fat cheese sauce made from cottage cheese and fat-free cheese powder; eating pasta with fat-free sauce for dinner three nights a week; using that slimy reconstituted butter powder on my veggies; buying low-fat everything; all that stuff.)

And I didn't lose one ounce. Oh, everything got firmer and higher, I looked a little better, and I felt a little better—I was fit, but fit and *fat*. I went to my wedding looking like a pretty little pale pink baby blimp. I bought new shorts to go on my honeymoon because all my old shorts were too small.

Well, by Labor Day, three months later, I had gained *another* ten or fifteen pounds. My *new* shorts were too small, and I was beginning to panic. Especially since my blood pressure was also up—borderline high for the first time in my life.

But I had been reading an old book on nutrition that I got at a used-book sale. It was by a fella named Gayelord Hauser, one of the first people to preach nutrition in this country—he worked for the old film studios, with stars like Greta Garbo. Back in 1952, Gayelord Hauser was saying something that was the opposite of what we've been told for the past twenty years: He said that obesity has *nothing* to do with overeating. He said that obesity is a *carbohydrate intolerance disease.*

I thought to myself, "Heck, nothing else is working! What do I have to lose?" I stopped eating high-carbohydrate foods—that is, starches and sugars—and *two days later* my shorts were loose. That was it! I cut back even further on carbs and started to read everything I could find on low-carb dieting.

Well! In two and a half weeks, I had lost ten pounds—eating eggs, meat, cheese, sour cream, real mayonnaise, and nuts.

Sounds insane, doesn't it?

But that wasn't all! I had also discovered that I felt *much* better on a low-carbohydrate diet. My energy level was higher and much more constant. I felt oddly clearheaded, and more positive, more emotionally resilient. Little things just didn't bug me anymore, and even big things were easier to shake off.

Hunger Gone!

Best of all, I wasn't hungry all the time anymore!

I had *always* been hungry before—I would have that nice, "healthy" breakfast of whole grain cereal and skim milk, and an hour and a half later, I could have eaten the *carpet,* I was so hungry! I'm not talking "head hungry"—I mean real, empty, growling stomach, getting tired hungry. I had often wondered why I was hungry all the time. I had read—and maybe you have, too—that if I ate a "healthy diet" (low in fat, high in carbohydrates) and "listened to my body," it would know how much food I needed. Unfortunately, I seemed to need enough for an entire army!

But on low carb, all of a sudden, I had a "normal" appetite. I could eat a cheese omelet for breakfast, and not be hungry again until *2:00 in the afternoon.* It was astonishing!

I even *forgot to eat* once or twice! My husband is a skinny thing with a light appetite, and he sometimes forgets to eat. When I first met him I could hardly believe that! I would say, "What, do you forget to breathe, too?" Now, I would come home intending to cook supper, but sit down to check my e-mail, and look up two hours later, saying, "Oh, yeah, I was supposed to cook...." For the first time in my life, I just wasn't emotionally involved with food.

Sometimes I'd even stop eating before I was done! That was astounding, too. I'm a charter member of the Clean Plate Club. If it's on that plate, it's MINE, and I'm gonna eat it. But all of a sudden, I'd be too full to finish sometimes, and push my plate away.

Well, I continued with the diet, ... I continued to lose weight, and to feel better. Eventually, I lost forty pounds, and lost most of that *without exercise*. I'm not knocking exercise. I do work out, and think it's very important. (You'll find a chapter on exercise later in the book.) But I think it's also important to note that I took four to five step aerobics classes a week without losing an *OUNCE* on my low-fat diet—but lost thirty-five pounds on low carb before I ever started working out again.

Am I a skinny girl now? No, I'm not. Last time I was tested, my body fat was at 26 percent, which is healthy, but not skinny-skinny. It is, however, considerably better than the 33 percent body fat that is average for American women my age. More important, the weight has stayed off, and *that's* what success looks like in the world of weight loss. More than 95 percent of people who lose weight gain it all back within three years. I'd rather lose forty pounds and keep them off, than lose sixty pounds and gain them back. And I bet you feel the same way!

Just as important, I've never felt better in my life! I have more energy at forty-five than I did at fifteen! Furthermore, my blood work—my cholesterol, blood pressure, all that jazz—is fantastic, despite the fact that heart disease runs in my family. (For those who want to know, at last testing, my cholesterol was 196, my triglycerides 80. My HDL, good cholesterol, was a magnificent 69, and my cholesterol/HDL ratio—supposed to be the most important thing—was 2.8. Anything under 4, so I'm told, is excellent. The nurses were stopping me in the hall, wanting to know what my secret was!)

Of course, I've told a lot of friends and family about this approach to eating. When you start losing weight, people come out of the woodwork, wanting to know how you did it. (Naturally, they're hoping the answer will be, "Why, I watched TV and ate potato chips, of course!" No such luck.) I told a lot of people about this way of eating before I wrote this book. And what happened?

My sister lost thirty pounds, and had to have all of her clothes taken in. As a bonus, her asthma improved! My friend Leslie lost twenty pounds using just *some* of the low-carb principles I taught her. One day at the drugstore, I spotted a total stranger about to buy those highly advertised diet shakes, and was pushy enough to tell him my story. When I ran into him a year later, I hardly recognized him—he'd lost seventy pounds, and had gone off his diabetes medication!

I went on a local cable access television program and gave a lecture that was the inspiration for this book. It became the most popular show in the history of the station, and I've gotten many phone calls from total strangers telling me that they saw the show, went low carb, lost weight, and improved their health. Over and over, I've seen this work.

I'm totally sold on low-carb dieting—and I'm convinced that, for many people, low fat/high carb is *worse than no diet at all*. In fact, it's gotten to the point that when I see people in the grocery store with that cart full of low-fat fake food, I want to run up to them and yell, "Don't do it, buddy! It's a lie, it's all a lie!" And that's why I've written this book. Low carb has changed my life, so much I just *have* to tell people about it.

Isn't This a Fad Diet?

"That's just a fad diet!" People throw that accusation at low-carb dieting. But let me ask those of you who are my age— forty-five—or older, a question: Don't you remember that when we were kids, everyone knew that if you wanted to lose weight, you gave up potatoes and spaghetti?

When I discovered that low carb was working beautifully for me, I read everything I could get my hands on about this subject: *Healthy for Life* and *The Carbohydrate Addict's Diet,* both by Drs. Richard and Rachael Heller, researchers at New York's Mt. Sinai Hospital; *The Zone,* by Barry Sears; *Protein Power,* by Drs. Michael and Mary Dan Eades, who have treated thousands of people for obesity at their clinic in Little Rock; and the well-known *Dr. Atkins' New Diet Revolution.* I came to understand the biochemical principles that make this diet work.

Maybe more interestingly, I found many *old* nutrition texts advocating low carb. For instance, *Calories Don't Count,* by Dr. Herman Taller, was fascinating. It was published in 1962. Dr. Taller got interested in low carb when one of his colleagues at the hospital suggested he try drinking polyunsaturated oil to lower his cholesterol. He started dutifully gulping six ounces of vegetable oil a day. Not only did his cholesterol drop—so did his weight! *And he'd added an extra 1,600 calories a day of pure fat!* Where does *that* fit into a low-fat diet?

I found *Eat Fat and Grow Slim,* by Dr. Richard MacKarness, with a preface by the wife of polar explorer Vilhjalmur Stefansson. Back in the twenties, Stefansson saw the Eskimo eating nothing but meat and fat, and thriving on it. He decided to see if a "civilized" man could do the same. He lived on only fresh meat and water for a year, while being monitored by physicians.

Not only did Stefansson not come down with scurvy or beriberi, he thrived. He came out of the experiment several pounds lighter, and with lower cholesterol, which was the only measure of cardiovascular fitness available back then. Later in life, in 1955, having grown a middle-aged paunch and suffering from a cerebral thrombosis, or blood clot, Stefansson went back on his Stone Age Diet, as he called it, with his wife joining him this time. The typical dinner in the Stefansson household, *according to Mrs. Stefansson,* was a steak and a cup of coffee, and occasionally half a grapefruit for dessert. They both lost weight. Stefansson had been slightly irritable and depressed but became his old ebullient, optimistic self again—and as a little, added bonus, his arthritis cleared up!

I even found an old diet book when I went to Vermont to help my mother settle her Aunt Betty's estate. We were clearing out her house when I found *Eat and Grow Thin*—a diet book from 1914, outlining—you guessed it—a low-carbohydrate program.

In fact, I learned that the *very first* mass-market diet book in the English language was published in 1852, and it was a *low-carbohydrate diet.* It was written by an Englishman named William Banting. How fat was William Banting? (*"How fat was he?"* I hear you cry.) He was so fat he had to walk down stairs backward, or he'd fall over. Doctors would tell him to eat less, and he'd try, but he'd be so awfully hungry that he just couldn't stick to it. (Sound familiar?) Then the doctors suggested exercise, so he went out and rowed on the Thames River every day—and it would make him so hungry, that he'd eat even more and gain weight. (Do you know this story?)

Finally, Banting went to a doctor because he was going deaf. The doctor looked in Banting's ears and discovered that Banting was going deaf because he had fat pressing on his eardrums! The doctor put Banting on a low-carb diet, and it worked! He lost weight. Banting was so pleased that he wrote a volume called *Banting's Letter on Corpulence,* and spent the money to publish it himself. It was a big success, and for a while in London in Victorian times, "banting" was the popular term for "dieting." Banting lived into his eighties, never regaining the weight.

What all of this told me is that, historically speaking, low carbohydrate is anything *but* a fad diet.

In retrospect, I should have known this. When I first got interested in nutrition, twenty-five years ago, I read Adelle Davis, who stressed the importance of protein and essential fats, and said that overweight people should avoid most carbohydrates, especially white flour and sugar. I also read *Psychodietetics,* by Drs. Cheraskin and Ringsdorf, who linked mental instability to a diet of sugar and other refined carbohydrates.

I gave up white flour and sugar completely, felt *so much* better, *and lost weight like crazy.* How I let myself be convinced a decade later that a big plate of white-flour pasta was health food, I'll never know, except... it's so seductive, isn't it? I don't know about you, but I *wanted* to believe. It was like telling an alcoholic that it is healthy to have a six-pack and a shot for dinner, or giving Dracula the key to the blood bank.

Now I know better. I know that a low-carbohydrate diet is medically sound and has withstood the test of time. And you'd have to pry my jaws open with a crowbar to get me to eat a high-carb meal again.

Another thing that convinces me that a low-carbohydrate diet isn't "fad dieting": It practically *forces* you to eat real food, with real nutritional value, rather than processed, chemical junk or nutritionless, refined white-flour products and sugary, ultra-processed cereals. Have you *looked* at the ingredients on some of those low-fat products? They don't come from a farm, they come from a lab! How can *anything* that has to be made in a factory be essential—or even beneficial—to human nutrition? It just doesn't make sense.

Let me give you an example. Here is a list of the ingredients in Paul Newman's Own Salad Dressing, Original Recipe. This is a dressing you may have been avoiding; after all, it has sixteen grams of fat per serving. However, it only has *one* gram of carbohydrate. Here's what's in it:

Olive oil, vegetable oil (soybean and/or canola oil), water, red wine vinegar, onion, spices, salt, garlic, lemon juice, distilled vinegar.

Sounds like food to me! You could whip this up in your own kitchen, if you wanted to. In fact, Paul started out making it in his basement.

Now, for contrast, here is the list of the ingredients in one of the most popular fat-free ranch dressings on the market (which, by the way, has eleven grams of carbohydrate per serving):

Water, corn syrup, cultured low-fat buttermilk (cultured lowfat milk), vinegar, sugar, cellulose gel, potato maltodextrin, xanthan gum with potassium sorbate, calcium sodium EDTA and sorbic acid as preservatives, propylene glycol alginate, phosporic acid, artificial color, natural flavor, monosodium glutamate, parsley, green onions, DL tocopherol acetate, spice, polysorbate 60, yellow #5.

What the heck is *that*? I'm not sure what propylene glycol alginate is, but it sounds suspiciously like antifreeze to me! Are we really supposed to believe that spicy corn syrup with unpronounceable chemicals is a wiser choice than olive oil and vinegar? You tell me which sounds like some bizarre fad!

Here's another example. A famous company makes both regular grated Parmesan cheese and fat-free fake Parmesan cheese. Here's what's in the real stuff:

Grated Parmesan cheese (part-skim milk, cheese culture, salt, enzymes), cellulose powder, potassium sorbate to protect flavor.

Okay, I'd rather they left out the preservative, but this is basically real food. (If you're curious, cellulose powder is just fiber; it's used to prevent caking.) But check out what's in the fat-free stuff:

Grated cheeses (Parmesan and Romano from cow's milk) (part-skim milk, cheese culture, salt, enzymes), starch, rice flour, enriched flour (durum wheat flour, thiamine mononitrate, riboflavin, niacin, ferrous sulfate), water, maltodextrin, cellulose powder, salt, and less than 2% whey, buttermilk, potassium sorbate as a preservative, glycerin, gum arabic, sodium phosphate, artificial color.

In other words, they've diluted the real, nutritious cheese with a bunch of refined starch and chemicals. Again, which sounds more like a fad food to you?

On a low-carb diet, we eat *real food,* the food that mankind has survived on for centuries: meat, poultry, fish, cheese, eggs, vegetables of almost every sort, nuts, seeds, olives, fresh natural oils, and real butter. How anyone who has been eating low-fat processed cold cereal and white flour bagels and low-fat, sugar-filled cookies and strange chemical salad dressings could think of these natural low-carb foods as a nutritional step *down* is beyond me.

CHAPTER TWO

So What Do You Eat?

WELL, WHAT I don't eat is at least three quarters of what you find in your grocery store. I don't eat bread, pasta, potatoes, rice, crackers, cereal, chips, dried beans such as kidneys or pintos, nothing thickened with flour or cornstarch, such as canned cream soups or jarred gravies. I also refrain from sugar, except for trace amounts in things like mayonnaise and Worcestershire sauce. No candy, cookies, cake, donuts, Danish (I do eat a little no-sugar-added ice cream now and then!); very little ketchup, steak sauce, or barbeque sauce (which have more sugar than ice cream!), etc. It may shock you to know that I also eat only a little fruit, and no fruit juice; they're high in natural sugars.

So what's left to eat!? Plenty!

Most days for breakfast, I have three fried eggs. For a change, I'll have a cheese omelet made with two or three eggs and jalapeno jack cheese—that's *real* cheese, not low-fat cheese—with salsa on top. Sometimes I have eggs scrambled with peppers, onions, and mushrooms, or four or five sausage patties, or a hamburger. If I'm eating out, hey, steak and eggs is always good! Hold the toast and hash browns, of course.

Lunches, if I'm eating at home, are usually tuna salad made with celery, peppers, and onion, with mayonnaise—again, *real* mayonnaise, not low-fat—or chicken salad with chopped pecans. Sometimes I'll make a protein shake, from a recipe I'll be sharing later on. If I'm having lunch out, I usually have a chicken Caesar salad, hold the croutons. If I'm going Mexican, I'll have fajitas. I'll skip the tortillas, pile the guacamole, sour cream, and pico de gallo right on top, and eat it with a fork. At the gyro joint, I get the meat, onions, sauce—all the insides of a gyro, without the bread—on top of a Greek salad. And extra olives. Fabulous!

Like everybody, sometimes I just catch some fast food. Most fast-food joints have some kind of grilled chicken salad, and I get these a lot. Sometimes I'll get a burger and a salad, instead. I'll put the hamburger patty, pickles, onions, all that stuff, on top of a garden salad, and eat them together. Pretty good! It's hilarious going into Burger King and ordering a Whopper, hold the bun. They *look* at you! You'd think I'd ordered roasted puppy on a stick or something. "Whaddaya mean, hold the bun?" What word didn't you *get*?

Since it's only my husband and me for dinner, we usually have a light meal—just a chop or a piece of chicken or a burger. Sometimes we have a salad or a vegetable, sometimes we don't. I make roasts fairly often—with just the two of us, they leave a lot of leftover meat to nibble on for days. Very convenient!

When I'm feeling creative and energetic, I make skillet cacciatore, with chicken and peppers and onions and tomato sauce and wine; or I make hamburger stroganoff, with lots of mushrooms and sour cream; or chicken paprikash, again, with lots of sour cream. I occasionally make cream soups—with real cream, not skim milk thickened with flour—or something really exotic, like tandoori chicken. On the other hand, sometimes I get pretty down-home and brown some pork sausage with onions and melt cheese over the top.

For snacks, I often eat nuts. I like pecans fried in butter, with ginger and soy sauce! I also love pumpkin and sunflower seeds, and these are usually available at convenience stores and truck stops. And I've created a sugar-free chocolate mousse that is to *die* for!

Sound good? It's pretty hard to feel sorry for yourself when you're eating this way!

CHAPTER THREE

Yikes! Sounds High Calorie!

I KNOW WHAT you're thinking: That stuff is loaded with fat! And fat is loaded with calories! How can I eat all that rich food and lose weight? And won't eating all that fat—all that saturated fat—make me a heart attack waiting to happen? Just how the heck does this work, anyway?

As a dieter, I'm sure you've heard that one pound of fat equals 3,500 calories. You've been told that you have to cut 3,500 calories from your weekly intake to lose one pound of fat. You've also been told that since fat has more calories per gram than anything else, if you cut the fat out of your diet, you'll lose weight, right? You've also been told that the opposite is true; that if you eat 3,500 extra calories in a week, you'll gain a pound. It sounds so easy, doesn't it?

A Calorie Is NOT a Calorie

There are only two problems with this. One, not all bodies are the same, and two, not all calories are the same.

"Oh, come on! A calorie is a calorie is a calorie!" That's what we've heard for years. And in one sense, that's true. A calorie is just a measure of energy—of fuel. Just as we buy fuel for our cars in gallons, we buy fuel for our bodies in calories. (By the way, that means that when ads say that their food is "loaded with energy," they mean "loaded with calories." Doesn't sound quite as good, does it? Any food that contains calories supplies energy.) Each calorie represents the same amount of energy, whether from fat, protein, or carbohydrate. It is true that if you eat 3,500 calories more than your body burns, you'll gain a pound of fat. If you eat 3,500 calories less than your body burns, you'll lose a pound of fat.

What calorie theory has missed, however, is that *foods have effects on the body separate from their calorie value.* What kind of effects? Dig this:

Back in the 1950s, two British doctors named Kekwick and Pawan did an experiment. They fed obese people a diet of 1,000 calories a day—a very low-calorie diet. The calories were the same; the *kind* of calories varied. And they found that on 1,000 calories a day of carbohydrate, most subjects lost very little weight. But when subjects were fed 1,000 calories a day of protein and fat, but *almost no carbohydrate,* they lost weight easily!

So Dr. Kekwick and Dr. Pawan conducted another experiment: They tried feeding their dieters 2,000 calories a day (sounds more comfortable to me!), in a "balanced diet"—meaning carbohydrate, along with protein and fat. The dieters didn't lose any weight, which won't come as any surprise to those of you who have struggled to lose weight at 1,200 calories a day, much less 2,000.

But here's the exciting part: When the doctors knocked the carbohydrate out of the diet, and fed their subjects a diet of protein and *fat,* they started losing weight! In fact, most of them found that so long as they didn't eat carbohydrates, they could eat *2,600 calories a day,* and still lose weight! Something was affecting the number of calories they burned.

So much for a low-fat diet.

By the way, Dr. Kekwick and Dr. Pawan aren't the only ones to have tested this. A fella named Dr. Frederick Benoit heard about their study and decided to check it out. Working at Oakland Naval Hospital in California, he tested seven men who weighed between 230 and 290 pounds.

First, Dr. Benoit put the men on a total fast—what we might call the no-calorie diet. If calorie theory is correct, this should have caused the fat to come off faster than anything, right? Wrong. They did lose weight, an average of twenty-one pounds in ten days. Sounds great! Except only seven and a half pounds, on average, was fat. The rest was water and *muscle*. Very bad news. They lost twice as much muscle as fat!

Then Dr. Benoit fed his obese men 1,000 calories a day—admittedly a very low calorie diet, but 1,000 calories more than they had been eating. Those 1,000 calories contained almost no carbohydrate, some protein, and a lot of *fat*. These guys were chowing down bacon, cream cheese, heavy cream, stuff like that. Guess what happened?

In a ten-day trial, they lost *twice* as much fat as they did eating *nothing at all!* An average of fourteen pounds of fat each. And they lost almost no muscle, just a half a pound apiece.

Much more recently, in 2000, a study was done at Schneider's Children's Hospital in New Hyde Park, New York, regarding obese adolescents. The kids were split into two groups, with one group eating a low-fat/high-carb diet, and one group eating a low-carb/high-fat diet. The low-carb group reported eating 66 percent *more* calories every day than the low-fat group—a total of 1,860 calories a day, as compared to just 1,100 calories a day for the low-fat kids. What happened?

The low-carb kids lost *twice* as much weight as the low-fat kids—and had a greater improvement in their triglycerides and HDL, to boot!

Are you beginning to wonder why you've been told to avoid fat? I sure am.

You can't eat unlimited calories on a low-carbohydrate diet. But you can eat enough calories so that you never have to be hungry again—and still lose weight.

Sound good?

Another Glitch in Calorie Theory
Then there's the other problem with calorie theory: It doesn't take individual differences in metabolism into account. Have you ever known someone who cannot gain weight no matter what they eat? I have a friend like this. His name is Tom. He's

6´6˝ and weighs about 160 pounds. He's muscular, but very, very thin. We used to date years ago, so I saw how he ate—we would go to an all-you-can-eat restaurant, and he would eat five full plates of food. When we got home, he'd eat a whole pint of Haagen-Daz. Just an hour later he'd be saying, "Do you think we should order a pizza?" Tom still eats this way. When we have him and his wife over, I have to cook for eight—and he's still just as skinny as can be now that he's forty.

Ever known someone like this?

Yet studies have shown that under some conditions, there are people who can *gain* weight on 1,000 calories a day! In fact, when I taught low-carb dieting at a local health club, one women said she had gained weight on *700 calories a day*, a starvation diet.

When people like Tom eat more than their usual intake of calories, medical studies have shown that their bodies simply crank up their metabolism and burn off the extra calories. The body adjusts the metabolism to the caloric intake. The person's temperature goes up very slightly, and they throw off the extra calories as heat—a process with the fancy name of "postprandial thermogenesis."

But those of us who fatten easily don't do this. Instead of burning off those extra calories, we store them instead; it's been called the "thrifty gene." And for centuries and centuries, this thrifty gene was a very, very good thing to have. If the crops had failed, you and I would have survived, and Tom would have died a painful death from starvation. We—you and I, the fat folks— we have *superior* bodies! *That's why there are so many of us!*

I want you to think about that for a minute. If, like me, you've been overweight most of your life, if you grew up dreading school every day because of how the kids would make fun of you, if you've gone to the beach in a T-shirt and cutoffs because you'd rather *die* than be seen in a bathing suit, you probably think of yourself as having a flawed body. Like you got a factory second or something. It's not true! *You have a superior body, a body that evolution favored!* Right now, I want you to stop thinking of yourself as third-rate goods. You got the good kind of body! You just live in the wrong *time and place*.

It's only because we have the incredible luck of living in an era and area where food is abundant all year long, year after year after year, that this genetic superiority is turned against us. Luckily, science is finally beginning to understand some of how those thrifty gene genetics work—and at the same time, learning why obesity is so very unhealthy, as well.

CHAPTER FOUR

But Aren't Carbs Essential?

Glucose, the sugar that your body burns as fuel, is a carbohydrate and is essential for a few organs in the body; the rest can run on fat, or on an alternate fuel called ketones, produced when your body burns fat for fuel without any carbohydrate. This sounds as if you have to eat at least some carbohydrate, right? (And all of the programs I'll outline for you do contain some carbohydrate, mostly in the form of vegetables. What we're avoiding here is concentrated carbohydrate foods: starches and sugars.)

But no, even though some glucose is essential, carbohydrate foods are not, for a very simple reason: Your body can turn protein, and to a much lesser degree, fat, into carbohydrate as it is needed—a process with the tongue-twisting name of gluconeogenesis, which means "making new sugar." And gluconeogenesis is, in many ways, a superior way to get glucose.

You've been told, no doubt, that you need carbs for energy. Yet after nearly twenty years of binging on pasta and bread and potatoes and fat-free cookies, fatigue is the single most common medical complaint in the country! Americans are just plain tired. The reason is simple, and lies in that old statement, that carbohydrates, and especially sugar, are "quick energy." Quick energy *sounds* good. But is it?

Let me ask you this: Would you burn straw in your wood stove to heat your house? Of course not. But straw is quick energy! And that's what's wrong with it, right? It burns *too* fast. If you wanted to burn straw for heat, you'd have to sit next to that wood stove and throw in another handful every three or four minutes. If you tried to put in a whole bale of straw, for lasting energy, it wouldn't work that way, would it? You'd burn the house down, because it still wouldn't burn gradually; it would all burn at once. In the same way, your body doesn't have any way to use carbohydrates gradually—except to store them as fat.

Or think of it this way: Gasoline is quick energy. *Really* quick energy! So quick that if you were to drop a lit match into your gas tank, it would burn so fast you'd be extremely fortunate to survive. The fact that gasoline is such quick energy is why cars have carburetors or fuel injectors—to make sure that only a tiny bit of gasoline gets lit at a time.

Your body doesn't have a carburetor. Your body doesn't have any way to feed the carbohydrate you eat into your bloodstream gradually. When you eat a breakfast of cereal, milk, juice, and sugar in your coffee, four sources of carbohydrate floods into your system fast. Very fast! Your body senses this as a threat, and takes action to fix it.

By the way, the *only* thing your body can use carbohydrates for is fuel. Protein can be used to make glucose for fuel, but it is also essential for body repair and maintenance, making enzymes, creation of antibodies to protect you from disease, all sorts of things. Fat can be used for fuel but is also used for making hormones, cell walls, nerve and brain tissue, useful things like that.

So here comes the million-dollar question: Why should a population that is sedentary and obese get most of their food as pure fuel? It makes no sense.

On a low-carb diet, your body rapidly remembers how to use fat—including your stored fat!—and protein for fuel. And it makes fuel out of fat and protein at the rate it needs it, not too slow, not too fast. The result? Energy that is stable and constant, instead of the roller-coaster ride from sugar break to sugar break.

Moderation?

"I believe in moderation in all things," people frequently tell me, implying, of course, that my avoidance of carbohydrate is immoderate, their intake of carbohydrate, including highly processed sugar and white flour, is moderate. I agree that moderation is a cardinal rule of health and happiness. One question, however, remains to be answered: What is "moderate"? Suppose, for instance, an individual were to eat only half of the sugar that the average American does. Sounds pretty moderate, doesn't it? Just think, only half!

Yet a person who ate only half the sugar of the average American would still be eating more than *ten times* the sugar that the average American ate in 1800, and more than four times the average American's sugar intake in post–Civil War times. *So what's moderate?*

If you were to drink *one* can of sugar-sweetened cola per day, and eat *no other sugar at all,* no cookies, no candy, no ice cream, no cold cereal, no prepared foods with added corn syrup, you would still be consuming well over *twice* the sugar that your Victorian era ancestors did. If you consumed a 1,500 calorie-per-day diet—a not-uncommon level among women—that one can of cola would represent fully 10 percent of your calories; one-tenth of your nutrients replaced with pure, valueless sugar. *So what's moderate?*

The explosion of American sugar consumption, from about 7 pounds per person per year in 1800 to an incredible 152 pounds per person per year now (and somebody's eating more, folks, because I'm eating less!), represents an increase of more than *2000 percent*, the single most drastic dietary change in the history of humankind.

The second most drastic change was the Agricultural Revolution itself, when humankind went from eating very few grains and beans, to making them the staples of the diet. To simply cut back "a bit" on these substances, and then call one's consumption "moderate," makes a joke of the very concept of moderation. In short, I *am* moderate. It is the standard American diet that is *desperately* immoderate.

CHAPTER FIVE

Okay, Explain How This Works

S O, HOW CAN I EAT fatty foods like meat and eggs and cheese and nuts, and not only lose weight, but improve my health? We've been told all these years that we need to lose weight to protect our health, because obesity will make us ill. It's no secret that fat people have more heart disease, high blood pressure, diabetes, and cancer than slim people. The assumption has been that obesity *causes* all these diseases.

Wrong! The latest research is beginning to make it clear that the reason obesity is associated with high blood fats, high triglycerides, high blood pressure, adult onset diabetes, and even the female cancers is *not* because obesity *causes* those problems, but rather because all of those problems *along with obesity* are symptoms of the same underlying problem—*carbohydrate intolerance disorder*, also referred to as *hyperinsulinemia* or *Syndrome X*. It all has to do with *insulin*—too much insulin.

What Does Insulin Do?

I'm sure you've all heard of insulin; it's that stuff diabetics have to inject. You may also know that those who are not diabetic produce insulin in their pancreas. But you probably don't really understand insulin's function in the body. It's really very simple—insulin's job is to take glucose (sugar) out of your bloodstream and move it into your cells. Period. Full stop.

Having a lot of sugar in your blood is very bad for you. [You see,] If it happens too often, for too long, you've got a disease we call *diabetes,* and it causes damage to blood vessels all over your body, and kills off pieces of you, bit by bit. It turns out that sugar sticks to proteins, and, in turn, makes them stick to each other inappropriately, making them stiffen up. This is called *glycation of proteins,* and it's the subject of the hottest antiaging research going on today. Diabetics have such high levels of sugar in their blood that this glycation of proteins happens at a terribly quick rate, destroying tissues all over their bodies.

So, when your body senses that your blood sugar level is high, it goes right into action, pumping out insulin to get that blood sugar back where it belongs. Insulin acts sort of like an usher or a doorman. It takes that sugar by the hand, and takes it to a special place on your cell, called an "insulin receptor." This is like a door for the sugar to go through. The insulin opens the door and waves the sugar to enter.

The first place the insulin takes the sugar to is your muscles. If you happen to be lifting weights or something, that's great! But what percentage of the time do you lift weights? For most of us sofa spuds, the muscles just aren't demanding that sugar. "What am I supposed to do with this?" the muscles ask. Then the insulin takes the sugar to your liver, and asks if it would like to store it as glycogen, a form of carbohydrate your body keeps in storage. But most of us already have as much glycogen as our bodies can handle.

So, the muscles don't want the sugar. The liver doesn't want the sugar. What to do with it now? Easy. The insulin opens the doors to your fat cells, and waves that sugar in, and the sugar is converted to fat in the process. Then, to make sure the stuff doesn't escape, the insulin slams the door shut, and *holds* it shut.

Insulin Stores Fat

Do you get what I'm saying? Insulin is what makes your body store calories as fat. And sugar—carbohydrate—in your blood makes your body produce insulin.

Now, this has some interesting implications. A hundred thousand years ago, this ability of insulin to cause fat storage was a very good thing. As I mentioned earlier, before mankind invented agriculture about 10,000 years ago, we didn't have access to large quantities of concentrated carbohydrates at all—most carbohydrates in a prehistoric diet came from vegetables—but there was considerably more carbohydrate available in the summer and fall, when the fruit was ripe. We ate carbohydrate, stored fat, and then had that fat available to get us through the long, cold winter.

But lack of food in the winter is not a big problem for most of us anymore—in fact, most of us do our best gaining from the end of November to the end of December, don't we? We eat large quantities of carbohydrates all year round, and store fat all year round, and we end up . . . well, round!

Here's the flip side of the fat-storage function of insulin: *Without insulin, you simply cannot store fat.* Period. Can't be done. Any juvenile onset diabetic knows this—one of the warning signs of juvenile onset diabetes is drastic weight loss. I knew a guy with this problem who told me that when his pancreas gave out, he lost twenty pounds in two days! *No fat storage without insulin.*

The Insulin Cycle
This knowledge gives us a powerful weapon in the fight against fat! If we can control insulin levels in our bodies, we can control fat storage. What causes insulin release? Rising blood sugar levels. What was happening to me, and what may be happening to you, is this. I would eat a big serving of carbohydrate—that whole grain cereal, or some pasta, or juice, whatever—and my blood sugar level would rise very quickly in response. Never forget that all carbohydrates are actually a form of sugar. Simple carbohydrates are the sweet sugars, such as table sugar and the sugar in fruit; "complex carbohydrate," another name for starch, means "a whole bunch of sugars linked together"—but chemically, they're all types of sugar.

So I'd eat those carbs, and my blood sugar would go shooting up—remember, the body has no way of absorbing the stuff gradually. My pancreas, seeing all that sugar in my blood, would say, "Hey, we have all this sugar floating around! Time to put that stuff away!" and it would release a big dose of insulin. The glucose in my blood would be marched right off to be stored as fat, and my blood sugar would drop drastically. Two things happened at the same time—I had a bunch of new fat in my fat cells (gee, what fun!), and I had no calories in my blood to use as fuel, so I got hungry and tired. I would eat more carbs—after all, carbs are low fat, and good for you!—and it would happen all over again. It was a vicious cycle: eat carbs, store fat, get hungry, eat carbs, store fat, get hungry.

But it was even worse than that. You see, medical research indicates that the more you go through this cycle, the more insulin your body releases. It's almost as if your pancreas gets panicky. "What?! *More* sugar? I thought I just got rid of this stuff! I'd better make a whole LOT of insulin!" And your blood sugar comes *crashing* down.

Are you beginning to understand why you're tired and hungry a lot of the time?

The Hunger Problem Gets Worse!

Ah, but there's more. You see, stable blood sugar is only one thing that makes you feel full and satisfied. Another thing that determines whether you feel full or hungry is a chemical with the tongue-twisting name cholecystokinin, which is why it's usually referred to as CCK. CCK is a chemical that is released by your brain in response to the right combination of foods, and makes you feel satisfied. In laboratory experiments, rats that were injected with CCK would sit in the midst of food and starve themselves, because they simply weren't hungry.

And what combination of foods causes your brain to release CCK? Certain amino acids, which are found in proteins, combined with *fat*. Without the fat and the protein—say, with a big plate full of pasta with fat-free sauce—you can eat and eat and *eat*, and *never* get filled up. Does this sound familiar?

Carbs Can't Fill You Up

This problem of crashing blood sugar, coupled with a lack of the foods needed to release cholecystokinin, is a huge weakness in low-fat/high-carb diet theory. After all, the whole point of a low-fat diet is to lower your overall calorie intake. Since fat has nine calories per gram, and protein and carbohydrates have only four calories per gram, the theory goes, if you cut out the fat, you could eat more food for fewer calories. And since carbohydrates are bulkier than proteins, and since many of the best protein foods also include fat, it looks like if you replaced those protein/fat foods with carbohydrates you could eat a huge pile of food and still lose weight.

The hitch is that Americans *have* dropped fat *as a percentage of our calories* a *lot*—25 percent overall. Guess what? We're eating *more* calories! And obesity is up by a whopping 30 percent! It's because we're eating a diet that is biochemically destined to *never fill us up*.

Here's a quick example of the power of a low-carbohydrate diet to quell hunger: A study published in the journal *Pediatrics* in 1999 looked at the effect of carbohydrates on hunger. Twelve obese teenage boys were fed one of three different breakfast and lunch meals. All the meals had the *exact same calorie count,* but one was full of high-impact carbs, one was full of low-impact carbs, and one was full of protein and fat, but very few carbs. Then the boys were allowed to eat at will for the rest of the day, and the amount of food they ate was tracked. What happened? The boys who had the high-protein, low-carb meals ate the least food of all. They simply weren't hungry later in the day. The boys who ate the low-impact carb meals ate 45 percent more. And the boys who ate the high-impact carb meals ate a whopping *81 percent more* during the afternoon than the boys who had eaten low carb.

Here Comes Addiction!

And now you can understand why carbohydrates, especially when eaten without protein or fat, are addictive. *They actually make you hungry!*

People talk about "food addiction"; it even has its own twelve step program, Overeaters Anonymous. But I don't know anyone who's addicted to food in general. I only know people who are addicted to carbohydrates.

Think about it. What do you binge on? What foods make you lose control? What foods do you crave?

Cookies? Sugar and starch.

Chips? Starch.

Ice cream? Sugar.

Bread? Starch.

Candy? Major sugar.

Do you like eggs? Do you enjoy a good steak? Does a fine cheese taste great? Of course! *Do you binge on them?* No. We enjoy these foods a great deal, but our hunger for them is finite. They fill us up. They satisfy us. We eat these foods *normally.*

But eating carbohydrates is like eating hungry pills. All the SnackWells in the world won't fill you up. They make you hungrier and hungrier and hungrier, until you start to wonder if you're crazy.

Aren't you tired of being hungry all the time? They tell you, eat low fat and control your portions.

I tell you that you will never be able to control your portions for the rest of your life if you are HUNGRY ALL THE TIME! I cannot think of anything more unnatural, more cruel, than telling people that they must sit in the midst of more food than any society has ever had available in the *history of the world,* and be *hungry.* No wonder people gain back their weight.

But you don't have to be hungry. I'm almost *never* hungry anymore. Certainly no one has ever been more carbohydrate addicted than I was, but I don't sit around going, "Oh, I wish I could have a potato, I wish I could have cookies, I wish I could have pasta." I can remember that those things tasted good—but somehow, I just don't care much anymore. That awful, driving hunger is *gone.*

You'll be astounded at how fast you can break the addiction cycle. Promise!

How carbohydrate addicted have I been? You might be tempted to think that I never really cared much about this stuff in the first place. Don't you believe it! When I was fourteen, I was stealing money from my parents to support my sugar addiction. I ate a half-pound Mr. Goodbar *and* a half-pound Hershey's bar with almonds on the way home from school every day. I also ate about a pound of lemon drops or five to six rolls of Wild Cherry Lifesavers during classes—sugar in my mouth every moment, all day long. I *also* ate three to five desserts in the school cafeteria at lunch every day. All of this in addition to whatever sugar I got in my meals at home. I had one *mean* monkey on my back!

When I was fifteen, I would start my school day with three or four chocolate donuts from the student store, washed down with three or four cups of vending machine cocoa. Because I was "watching my weight," I would have a chocolate milkshake for lunch instead of real food. What I remember most vividly from that year is wandering around my high school, muttering, "I'm so tired! I'm soooo tired!" Dead on my feet at fifteen—from "energy food."

CHAPTER SIX

Insulin Doesn't Just Make You Fat and Tired

B
UT OBESITY'S NOT the whole story. You see, medical research is beginning to link high levels of insulin with all sorts of other health problems—high cholesterol, high triglycerides, high blood pressure, adult onset diabetes, polycystic ovarian syndrome (PCOS), and the female cancers. There's even some evidence, which we'll discuss later, showing high levels of insulin may increase pain and inflammation and weaken your immune system.

High Blood Pressure
High levels of insulin in your blood will cause your kidneys to hold on to sodium. You've probably heard that sodium is what you're supposed to avoid if you have high blood pressure. But you may not have heard that for the vast majority of people, a low-sodium diet doesn't improve their blood pressure at all. It turns out that for many people, the problem is not that they're getting too much sodium in their diet, but rather that because of the insulin in their blood, their kidneys are hanging on to too much sodium, and thus hanging on to too much water, with high blood pressure as a result. You can take diuretics—water pills— or you can control your insulin levels, and lose the extra sodium, and the extra water with it.

You remember that I mentioned that on low fat/high carb my blood pressure was borderline high for the first time in my life? It normalized within a couple of weeks on this diet, probably because, for the most part, the first five or ten pounds I lost were water. I didn't sleep much for the first few days—too busy going to the bathroom!

(By the way, some critics say you *only* lose water on low carb, to which my response is: *FIVE GALLONS?!* I've lost *FIVE GALLONS* of water?! I doubt it, but if I've lost that much water, I'm sure glad to be rid of it!)

Heart Disease

If Americans know one thing, it's that fat and cholesterol will give you heart disease. Cholesterol is practically a poison, for heaven's sake!

No, it's not. Believe it or not, cholesterol is an *essential part of your body chemistry!*

First of all, your brain and your nerves have high levels of cholesterol. Sounds pretty important right there! Many of your hormones are made from cholesterol, including your sex hormones. It's cholesterol in your skin that turns to vitamin D in the sunlight. And cholesterol is essential for the walls of every cell in your body.

Indeed, if your cholesterol levels are too *low*, you're at an increased risk of death from all sorts of things, but especially from cancer. You read that right—low cholesterol, under about 170, is a risk factor for cancer, and the lower it gets, the greater your risk. Low cholesterol also increases your risk of some kinds of stroke. Furthermore, low cholesterol appears to cause depression, and in middle-aged-to-elderly men, it's a strong risk factor for—believe it or not—death from violence and/or suicide!

Lower is *definitely* not always better where blood cholesterol is concerned.

In fact, cholesterol is so important that if you stop eating it, your body makes more. More than two-thirds of the cholesterol in your body is made *by* your body, and if you stop eating cholesterol, your body simply increases production to make up the difference. If you eat more, your body makes less.

That is, unless something messes up the balance mechanism. What can do that? *Insulin!* Insulin actually makes it harder for your body to take cholesterol out of your bloodstream and move it into the cells where your body uses it. Since your body knows only how much cholesterol it has in its cells, *not* how much it has in its bloodstream, it thinks it's not getting enough. Your body then goes to work making cholesterol! This tendency of insulin to inhibit the retrieval of cholesterol from the blood is quite enough to cause dangerously high cholesterol all by itself.

If you lower your level of insulin, your body can get access to the cholesterol in your bloodstream. It calms down, stops making too much cholesterol, and starts using up the excess in your blood. The result? Your LDL, or "bad" cholesterol, drops! That is, if you're one of the many, many people for whom insulin was the whole problem in the first place.

Which explains an article in *Southern Medical Journal* in January 1988. Dr. H. L. Newbold was treating a group of people who had serious food allergies. He found that most of them could eat beef without trouble. So he told them to eat steaks with plenty of fat—and other meat if they could tolerate it—plus a few raw veggies and a little fruit. Guess what? The average patient's cholesterol *dropped* from 263 to 189! Further, their HDL (good cholesterol) was going up, while their bad LDL cholesterol was going down.

Far more recently, in 2002, a study was done at Duke University. Conducted by Dr. Eric Westman, who presented the results to a stunned audience at an American Heart Association annual meeting, the study compared the results of the very low-carb, high-fat Atkins diet and the American Heart Association's low-fat "Step 1" diet. Westman had studied 120 overweight volunteers, who were randomly assigned to one diet or the other. Six months later, the results were compared.

The upshot? First of all, more volunteers had stuck with the Atkins diet than with the low-fat diet—I'm guessing because it didn't call for them to be hungry all the time. This, in itself, is a big deal, since livability is a *major* part of long-term weight loss success.

Better yet, the Atkins dieters had lost an average of thirty-one pounds apiece, compared with an average of twenty pounds apiece for the Step 1 dieters. That's more than 50 percent greater weight loss!

But what *really* stunned the skeptics was that the Atkins dieters had a *greater* improvement in their blood work, and a *greater* theoretical reduction in heart attack risk! Both groups had a modest drop in total cholesterol. But the Atkins dieters had a 49 percent drop in triglycerides, while the low-fat dieters' triglycerides dropped only 22 percent—and triglycerides are considered one of the most powerful heart disease risk factors. Furthermore, *only* the Atkins dieters had an increase in HDL "good" cholesterol, a very protective factor.

The problem is *not* cholesterol in your diet. Think about it: Beef is high in cholesterol, right? Cows are vegetarians! They eat grass, and on modern farms are fed a lot of grain—the same low-fat, high-carb grain you've been told to eat to be healthy. *So where does the cholesterol come from?* It comes from the cow's own body, which has been fooled by insulin into thinking the cow needs more cholesterol!

Certainly, my cholesterol is *great* after eight years of feasting on fat while avoiding grains and other carbs. And I've seen the same thing happen to many other people. *However!* This does not seem to work for everybody. There is a minority of people who, when they go on a low-carb diet that includes lots of fatty red meat, egg yolks, cream and butter, and other sources of saturated fat, have a sort of 50/50 reaction: Their triglycerides come down, and their good cholesterol (HDL) goes up, which is fine; but their bad cholesterol (LDL) and total cholesterol go up, as well, which is not so good.

No one is quite certain why this should be so; the simple, basic answer, no doubt, is that people are different, and there's more than one cause of cholesterol troubles. The Eades feel that some people are sensitive to a chemical called arachidonic acid, which often is found in tandem with cholesterol and saturated fat. Dr. Atkins felt that a minority of the population is sensitive to saturated fats (NOT to cholesterol in the diet. Oddly enough, there is very little evidence that eating cholesterol causes high cholesterol in anybody.).

Either way, the solution is the same. If you have cholesterol trouble, get tested a few months after going on your low-carb diet, and see where you stand. (This presupposes that you know where you stand *before* you go on the diet! If you don't, take care of that little matter right away. Otherwise, when you get tested after having been on the diet for a while, you'll have no idea whether those numbers, no matter what they are, represent an improvement, or a worsening, of your health.) Keep in mind that the numbers are *not* as important as the *ratios;* if your LDL and total cholesterol have gone up a little, but your HDL has gone up a *lot,* and your triglycerides have come down, you may actually be at lower risk, even though the numbers look worse at first glance. And remember that total cholesterol can actually be too *low.* You're shooting for a total cholesterol number of between 170 and 220.

Be *very* aware that the most important thing is the ratios, *not* your total cholesterol number! My friend Mary, who had been on a basic low-carb diet, called me in a panic one day because she'd just gotten her blood work, and her total cholesterol number had jumped quite a lot. (Her total cholesterol had always been in the range we now know to be too low, although no one ever told Mary that.) However, when we looked at her ratios— total cholesterol/HDL, triglycerides/HDL, LDL/HDL—it turned out that Mary had a *remarkably* low risk of heart disease; her HDL was *very* high, and her triglycerides were very, very low. (Since we had no idea what her LDL/HDL breakdown or triglycerides had been when her total cholesterol was so low, we have no idea if she's healthier or not—but it would be hard to have better ratios than Mary has now.)

How do you work those ratios? Easy. Get a copy of your blood work (it must be "fasting blood work" to be accurate regarding triglycerides) and a simple pocket calculator. Divide your total cholesterol number by your HDL number; the result should be 4 or below. Then divide your LDL by your HDL; if you're a man, a result of 3.55 gives you average risk, anything below that is better. If you're a woman, 3.22 gives you an average risk, anything below that is better. And for perhaps the most important ratio, divide your triglycerides by your HDL; anything less than 2 is good. These three numbers should give you a clear idea of where you stand, in terms of risk of heart disease.

If it turns out that you are in the minority whose ratios worsen on a low-carb diet with unrestricted saturated fat intake, what do you do? Well, first of all, you *don't* go back to a low-fat/high-carb diet—you'll lose the beneficial HDL and triglyceride levels you've been achieving. Instead, you take care to improve the balance of *types* of fat in your diet. This means choosing lean meats and trimming the fat, eating more fish and poultry, throwing away every other egg yolk (you could eat egg substitutes instead, but I think they taste nasty, I'm suspicious of the chemicals in them, and they cost an arm and a leg), perhaps choosing reduced-fat cheeses and sour half-and-half instead of sour cream.

Also make sure you've eliminated "hydrogenated vegetable oils"—margarine and vegetable shortening—from your diet *completely*. This will include ruling out just about all commercially deep-fried foods; almost invariably these are fried in hydrogenated oils. But then most deep-fried foods are breaded, so you shouldn't be eating them anyway! Regular-Joe type peanut butter, such as Skippy and Jif and Peter Pan, is loaded with hydrogenated oils. (Sugar, too!) Peanuts are okay for low carbers, in moderation, but if you want peanut butter, buy natural peanut butter, the kind with oil on top. (That's why the manufacturers hydrogenate the oil in most peanut butter, to keep it from rising to the top.) The unnatural saturated fats created by the hydrogenation process, called *trans* fats, are far more damaging than any naturally occurring saturated fat.

At the same time, increase your intake of fish—shoot for at least three fish meals a week, more won't hurt—and of healthy fats, like olive oil and olives, raw nuts and seeds. If you really dislike fish, you might consider taking EPA supplements, either from fish oil or from flax seed. These can have a very beneficial effect on cholesterol.

Supplements of GLA (another healthy oil), from either evening primrose oil or borage oil, have also been shown to help lower cholesterol. Capsules of both these oils can be found at any health food store. Soluble fiber helps some people; you might take a fiber supplement—just be sure that it's sugar-free. Better yet, take flax seed meal—the combination of EPAs and soluble fiber in flax is a great one-two punch for lowering total cholesterol. Niacin—vitamin B3—has been clinically proven effective for lowering cholesterol, but needs to be handled with care. Also, be sure you're taking a good, broad-spectrum multiple vitamin and mineral supplement. More about both of these later.

All of this should do the trick!

Depression and Mental Illness

Have you noticed how many people seem to be depressed these days? It seems to me that there are a whole lot of folks these days who have no real definable problems, and yet are miserable and anxious a lot of the time. Sometimes I think everybody but me is on Paxil!

Now, I'm not going to tell you that a low-carbohydrate diet will cure all mental illness. The brain is an incredibly complex organ, and there's no one answer to all mental problems. There are some very real chemical imbalances for which antidepressant drugs and other medications are nothing short of a miracle and a blessing. Furthermore, if you've had a lot of serious emotional trauma in your life, I'm not sure there's any biochemistry that will fix it, just like that.

On the other hand, *your brain is a part of your body.* It amazes me how many people don't seem to realize that! I mean, we all know that if we put alcohol in our mouths, it affects our brains; if we put a joint in our mouths, it affects our brains; if we put pills in our mouths, it affects our brains. But it doesn't seem to occur to us that the food we put in our mouths affects our brains! *Yet, our brains can be only as healthy as our bodies.* The brain is *just* as dependent on the food we eat as any other organ is; maybe more so. Is it any wonder that a country that lives on sugar, white flour, and chips is having trouble with mental illness right along with physical illness?

So where does carbohydrate intolerance fit into this picture? Unstable blood sugar, *exactly* the blood sugar swings I just described, is enough to cause mental illness *all on its own*. Here's a list of the most common mental symptoms of low blood sugar, properly called *hypoglycemia*:

Nervousness
Irritability
Exhaustion
Faintness, dizziness, weak spells
Depression
Headaches
Mental confusion
Insomnia— especially going to sleep, then waking up
   after an hour or two and lying awake feeling anxious
Internal trembling—feeling shaky inside, while your
   hands are steady
Anxiousness—constant worry about nothing in particular
Trouble concentrating

Quite a list, huh? And one that would send a lot of people straight to the doctor, and then to the pharmacy. But all of these symptoms can be cleared up by a diet that stabilizes blood sugar, *if* (and *only* if) *blood sugar swings are causing them in the first place.*

With America chowing down on a diet practically *designed* to destabilize blood sugar, is it any surprise that we're seeing a huge increase in antidepressant prescriptions? *I would lay the bill for the antidepressant explosion of the 1990s directly at the doorstep of the low-fat theory of the 1980s.*

Another interesting new tidbit is the research that is starting to connect cholesterol to mental health. As I mentioned, there's a strong correlation between very low blood cholesterol levels— under 160—and depression, violence, and suicide. This does *not* necessarily mean that low blood cholesterol causes mental illness; mental illness of some kinds may cause low cholesterol. Or some third factor may be causing both. The research is inconclusive. But there is evidence that cholesterol is involved in regulating your brain's level of *serotonin,* a chemical that makes us feel cheerful and calm, the very chemical that Prozac, Paxil, and the other recent antidepressants are designed to increase. Pass those eggs!

Here's another problem with the low-fat/high-carb diet as most Americans eat it: It robs the body of B vitamins. All carbohydrates require B vitamins to be processed in your body, but *only* whole grain, unrefined carbohydrates contain enough B vitamins for their own metabolization. If you eat a lot of white flour and sugary low-fat stuff (or sugary high-fat stuff, for that matter!), your body will take the B vitamins from the good stuff you eat to process the refined junk.

Why is this so important? Because *all* of the B vitamins include mental problems among their deficiency symptoms. If you get deficient enough, you'll literally go insane. It's unlikely to go that far, but lower-level deficiencies can make you anxious, irritable, jittery, even paranoid. (Vitamin B deficiencies can also make you tired, which is pretty depressing in its own right.)

A low-carb diet stops this B vitamin drain on your body and contains most of the B-rich foods, including meat (especially organ meats), eggs, nuts, seeds, and peanuts.

Is a low-carbohydrate diet *guaranteed* to cure *all* depression and other mental ills? No, of course not. But it will help many, many people. And the wonderful thing is that it's both free and harmless to find out if it will help *you*! One of the most common remarks I hear from low-carb dieters is how much more cheerful they feel—when most diets make you feel cranky!

In fact, I know of at least one person who had a very low carbohydrate diet prescribed by their psychiatrist as a treatment for depression. Closer to home, I have one member of my immediate family who got off of Prozac using a low-carbohydrate diet and nutritional supplements, and feels better than he ever did on the drug. And a dear friend of mine—who, by the way, is not overweight by any stretch of the imagination—is an adult victim of child abuse, suffering from depression and attention deficit disorder. Despite being very slim, he has found that keeping his blood sugar stable by avoiding large amounts of concentrated carbohydrate and eating plenty of protein is *instrumental* to maintaining balanced mental function. He feels better than he ever has. That's not too shabby for a program most people use to lose weight!

Kinda gives a new meaning to "A sound mind in a sound body," doesn't it?

Diabetes

After years and years of the insulin cycle, many people start to lose the ability to use insulin properly. With all that abuse, the areas on the cells that use insulin, those insulin receptor sites, start to malfunction. It's like the hinges on the door start to wear out. This is called "insulin resistance." Your body churns out even MORE insulin to get the sugar out of your blood and into fat storage. If this continues, you start to have both high insulin levels and high sugar levels in your blood, and eventually you'll develop adult onset or type II diabetes. Now, along with the damage caused by high levels of insulin, you also have the damage caused by high blood sugar levels. Very bad news indeed.

I've talked to a woman who actually gave herself adult onset diabetes by eating a low-fat/high-carb diet. (She didn't lose much weight, either!) So long as she sticks to her low-carbohydrate diet, her blood sugar is normal, and she needs no medication. Pretty cool!

You need to know that since America went low fat, type II diabetes has skyrocketed. And the number of diabetics worldwide is predicted to double *again* between now and 2025. Some researchers think it's just because the population is getting older. But guess what? This disease, traditionally called "adult onset" diabetes, is now growing rapidly in American *children*. Think that might have to do with the fact that the average American kid gets *half* his calories from sugar, and a whole bunch more from white bread, canned pasta, and chips, hmmm?

You don't want diabetes. It's an incredibly ugly disease. It can give you heart disease, make you blind, make your fingers and toes die one by one, and cause impotence in men. If you suspect your blood sugar is unstable, take the warning and do something about it *now*.

Cancer

Then there's cancer. Women, in particular, have been told to fear breast cancer from a diet high in fat. It is true that women who are obese have a higher risk of breast cancer than women who are not. Because of this, it has been assumed that a low-fat diet will prevent breast cancer, just as it has been assumed that a low-fat diet will cure obesity. Wrong!

It will amaze and reassure you to hear about the Harvard Nurses Study. This is a HUGE study—90,000 nurses were included, and they've been studied for more than a decade, which is almost unprecedented in scope. The researchers divided the nurses into five groups by their fat intake. The group with the *lowest* fat intake had the *highest* rate of breast cancer! Haven't read about that lately, have you?

In February of 1998, the *New England Journal of Medicine* published an article in which the statistics from seven different studies of the effect of a low-fat diet on breast cancer were analyzed. Guess what? There was *no* evidence that a low-fat diet decreased the risk of breast cancer. In fact, the statistics indicated that a very low-fat diet *increased* the risk of breast cancer.

It's also interesting to note that the first formula for predicting cancer risk in populations was presented in a medical paper in 1843, by a fellow named Stanislaw Tanchou—and it was based on grain consumption. The more grain a given population ate, overall, the more cases of cancer could be found. This is echoed by a 1996 study reported in the highly respected medical journal, *The Lancet*, that examined breast cancer rates in Italian women. The study showed a *decreased* risk of cancer associated with *increased* fat intakes (no doubt that healthy Italian olive oil), and an *increased* rate of cancer associated with an increased consumption of *carbohydrate*.

How about colon cancer? For a long time it's been considered axiomatic that a low-fat, high-fiber diet was the way to prevent colon cancer. Turns out it's not true.

In the April 19, 2000, issue of the *New England Journal of Medicine,* there appeared two separate large studies regarding the effect of a low-fat, high-fiber diet for preventing colon cancer. Both studies showed *no* benefit whatsoever.

The studies were done at the National Cancer Institute, and the University of Arizona, respectively. The NCI study involved having 1,905 people eat various diets for four years, and then counting the precancerous growths in their colons. (Now *there's* a job I don't want . . .) The U of A study involved 1,303 patients, and a trial of a diet heavy in wheat bran cereal. This study also looked at the occurrence of precancerous growths, or polyps, rather than cancers themselves. Precancerous polyps can readily be removed. Untreated, about 5–10 percent of them will turn cancerous within ten years.

The researchers in these two studies suggested that a low-fat, high-fiber diet could conceivably act on colon cancer in later stages of development, or if eaten for a much longer period of time. But they also admitted that there's no hard evidence of this.

I found both revealing and amusing a quote from Dr. Arthur Schatzkin, of the National Cancer Institute. "It was very disappointing," he said. "A positive result would have been a very strong statement." A very strong statement of *what*? That the medical establishment hasn't been leading us in the wrong direction for the past twenty years? I thought that the point of medical research was to find useful information, not to "make a strong statement." It's clear that Dr. Schatzkin "knows" that a low-fat diet is the "healthiest" diet, and he isn't about to let a little thing like research get in his way.

More to the point, Dr. Tim Byers, from the University of Colorado School of Medicine, said, "There may be many reasons to eat a diet that is low in fat and high in fiber, fruits, and vegetables...but preventing colorectal adenomas...is not one of them."

In July of 2000, another new report was presented to the Society for Epidemiologic Research at their annual meeting in Seattle, Washington. What did it say? That consumption of nonfiber carbohydrates—that is, the usable, absorbable carbs that I'm suggesting you avoid—*increases the risk of colon cancer.*

The study was done at the University of British Columbia and involved analyzing data on the consumption of carbohydrates by 490 "migrant Chinese" who had colorectal cancer, and comparing their diets with those of 1,100 healthy migrant Chinese who served as controls. All subjects were between ages forty and eighty and were living in North America, which is, I assume, where the "migrant" part comes in.

The researchers adjusted for age, saturated fat intake, fiber intake, calcium consumption, body mass index, level of exercise, and family health history, and came to the conclusion that, overall, the folks who ate the most digestible carbohydrates had a greater risk of colon cancer than those who ate the least. I do not know if any of those folks were on a diet as low in carbs as most low-carb dieters eat.

Interestingly, the risk was much different for men than for women, both in degree—women with the highest carbohydrate consumption had more than *seven times* the risk of those with the lowest, while men had only double the risk—and in the location of the cancers—women had a higher risk for cancer in the right colon, men, in the left colon. Either way, this study represents another nail in the coffin of the failed low-fat/high-carb diet theory.

I will wait with great interest for more studies to be done.

While we're on the subject, how many of you have been told that while the origin of most cancers remains a mystery, we do know for certain what food it is that cancers feed on: SUGAR. Would you like to starve any potential cancers in your body? Try a low-carbohydrate diet. In fact, I've read about a few medical studies where ketogenic diets—the very lowest carbohydrate, highest fat sort of diets—have been shown to slow and even *reverse* tumor growth, in animals and in pediatric cancer patients, by limiting the glucose available to feed the tumor. At the same time, these diets avoid the terrible wasting that comes with cancer, by providing calories as *fat*—which the healthy tissues can use as fuel, but the cancer can't.

Polycystic Ovarian Syndrome

Ever heard of polycystic ovarian syndrome, also called PCOS? You will.

Polycystic ovarian syndrome has only recently been identified, and there are many doctors who are still not up to speed on the symptoms of the syndrome, so it is important that women become informed. What gives PCOS its name is ovarian cysts. A cyst is a small, fluid-filled sac, sort of like a blister. There are several types of cysts, some quite normal—just a part of the ovulatory cycle—and some that can grow and even become cancerous over time, and must be removed. The "polycystic" in the name of PCOS means that the ovaries grow a lot of cysts, sometimes becoming quite full of them. This can cause pain, and can also cause irregular periods and fertility problems.

PCOS is not simply a gynecological problem, it is a full-body, systemic metabolic disorder with some *very* serious side effects. The underlying cause of PCOS is severe insulin resistance—the inability for insulin to enter the cells, just like we talked about in the section on diabetes. This means that if you have PCOS, you are at a high risk for all the health problems that go along with serious hyperinsulinemia—high blood fats, high blood pressure, heart disease, and type II diabetes. You are also at increased risk of breast cancer, and because PCOS messes up your menstrual cycle, there's some suspicion that it also increases your risk of endometrial cancer. We're talking serious stuff, here.

Those high levels of insulin in turn cause the ovaries to make too much testosterone. (Yes, women have testosterone, too. We're just supposed to have less than men do.) Those high levels of testosterone can cause irregular menstrual periods, infertility, facial hair growth, acne, and thinning hair—a sort of "male pattern baldness" in women. Obesity is usually a part of the picture as well, and can make matters worse, because stored body fat can itself affect levels of circulating hormones. Indeed, women with PCOS have runaway levels of estrogen, too.

The overall symptom pattern of PCOS includes:

Irregular periods

Infertility

Acne
Facial hair growth
Thinning head of hair
Ovarian pain
Obesity, especially abdominal obesity

If you have several of these symptoms, or if you have irregular periods (defined as six or fewer periods a year), you should see your doctor. If you have a daughter with some or all of these symptoms, be aware that PCOS can start quite young. I have here in front of me a medical journal article titled "Early metabolic abnormalities in adolescent girls with polycystic ovarian syndrome." It details a study done on girls with PCOS who were all of twelve years old. Get the kid to a doctor and on a low-carb diet *now,* and prevent years of trouble.

The doctor should *not* just do an ultrasound to look for ovarian cysts; many women have ovarian cysts and do not have PCOS. To diagnose PCOS, your doctor should look at your menstrual history and do extensive blood tests, looking at levels of glucose, HDL and LDL cholesterol, triglycerides, and especially testosterone and other sex hormones.

Once diagnosed with PCOS, a low-carbohydrate diet becomes *vital,* because it will lower the levels of insulin in your bloodstream, which will, in turn, lower your body's runaway production of testosterone. The weight loss that a low-carb diet brings is also helpful, since simple weight loss, however achieved, appears to lessen insulin resistance, which, in turn, lowers blood insulin levels even more. According to the articles I was able to find on the subject—both popular press articles and medical journal stuff—by lowering insulin levels and causing weight loss, a low-carb diet *by itself* has been sufficient for some women to start menstruating again and become pregnant. That's pretty impressive.

Exercise is also important, since it is also a good way to increase insulin sensitivity. (Yes, this means *you.* Go for a walk, and lift some weights—resistance exercise appears to be more effective than aerobic exercise for improving insulin sensitivity.)

However, PCOS is a nasty and potentially *very* dangerous thing, and I would NOT advise—if you recognize these symptoms in yourself—that you simply go on a low-carb diet, lose some weight, and call it quits at that. You're playing games with your life, here. It is VERY IMPORTANT that your doctor monitor you. If your doctor doesn't understand PCOS, FIND ANOTHER DOCTOR.

There are some drug treatments that help PCOS. You may be put on drugs that increase insulin sensitivity, the same drugs usually used for diabetics. Make sure that your doctor understands that you also plan to eat a low-carbohydrate diet, so that he or she doesn't prescribe more insulin-lowering drugs than you need.

However, some drug treatments are turning out to be a not-so-great idea. In particular, birth control pills are often prescribed because they help with acne and facial hair. However, studies show that women who take birth control pills for PCOS are more likely to become diabetic, which is *not* what you want. Eat your low-carb diet, exercise regularly, and be patient!

There is no complete cure for PCOS at this time; indeed, it isn't even well understood, nor are we certain how many women have PCOS, although estimates run as high as 10 percent of the female population (!). The good news is that a low-carbohydrate diet, coupled with help from a knowledgeable physician, should help you prevent many of the most devastating health consequences of PCOS. A low-carb diet can also help you lose some of the excess weight that comes with PCOS, and that is very good news indeed, since in many women a loss as modest as 10 percent of body weight is enough to regularize periods and allow them to become pregnant.

Alcoholism

Another health problem that appears to be strongly tied to carbohydrate intolerance is alcoholism. The connection isn't completely clear, but what information I could find is very interesting!

When I first got interested in nutrition, *everybody* was recommending a high-protein diet, with no refined carbohydrates.

Back then, I read accounts of alcoholics being treated successfully with high-protein/low-carb diets. At the time, I had no way of evaluating these claims, but I knew that nutrition had greatly improved *my* mental state. So I stashed the information away in the mental file labeled "Points to Ponder."

Since rediscovering low-carbohydrate dieting, I've gone back to look at some of those old claims. Here are a couple of interesting quotes:

> "*All* alcoholics are hypoglycemic, for it is an inevitable result of substituting whiskey for food. Some alcoholics *begin* by becoming hypoglycemic, and at the point where the low blood sugar would ordinarily cause a craving for sweets; they pervert the craving into an appetite for alcohol. *That* group in the alcoholic population can be *cured* of alcoholism by adopting and staying on the hypoglycemia diet.... This paragraph is *not* based on theory. Let me quote from one of hundreds of letters: 'I didn't make any vows, pledges, promises. I didn't ask for the intervention of the Almighty, and I did no praying. I didn't call on fellow alcoholics or ex-drinkers for aid. I had already been through A.A., Antabuse, shock treatment, and psychotherapy without results. I just went on the hypoglycemia diet, and a few months later, suddenly realized two things: I hadn't had a drink in weeks, and I didn't want one.'"

(*New & Complete Nutrition Handbook: Your Key to Good Health,* Carlton Fredericks, Ph.D., 1976.)

The other story is very long, but striking. It starts by talking about the writer's childhood diet:

> "My parents were opposed to drinking. Liquor (even beer and wine) was unknown in our home. But our patterns of living and eating predisposed each of the children in that family to a life of alcoholism or some other form of addiction . . . We never—or almost never—ate breakfast. On Saturdays, Sundays, and holidays some of

us had breakfast—a breakfast that was always cereal, sugar, pancakes loaded with carbohydrates, or waffles with maple syrup. But on weekdays, we went off to school with no breakfast. Lunch . . . if we were at the school cafeteria, we invariably chose foods that were high carbohydrate: potatoes, pasta, desserts, sweet rolls.... Desserts were not only served at every meal, but also candy and cookies were always available at any time of day. We ate lots of this kind of food."

The writer goes on to describe his descent into alcoholism, to the point where "During one period of great stress, I found that I was drinking my lunch and drinking all afternoon and evening as well. Soon a drink was essential to get me started in the morning; my hands trembled uncontrollably without it. I still ate no breakfast, for the drink took the place of it." However, eventually, the writer went to work in a medical library, and started reading the publications that came across his desk. "I began to read about alcoholism; I began to read about diet. I had access to all the literature I needed on both subjects, and so I began to change my way of eating. I ate eggs for breakfast, and I was astonished at the stability and feeling of well being this single item of food brought me.... The results were remarkable. I could get along without a drink at mid-morning. And I forced myself to eat a high-protein lunch—lots of meat, cheese, milk. I found that I could get through the afternoon without a drink—if I had a 4 o'clock snack of cheese, peanuts, or some other high protein food."

The writer continued to improve his nutritional status, adding supplements and increasing his protein intake still further. "Dinner consisted of almost nothing but high-protein foods—meat, fish, poultry, eggs, cheese— and almost no carbohydrates. Snacks were always high protein. The vitamins and the high protein meals became a way of life. And I found that I no longer had the almost constant craving for alcohol."

He finally says, "I call myself a cured alcoholic. I know that experts in this field declare positively that there is no such thing—that the true alcoholic can never take a drink again if he wants to remain sober. So, perhaps, I am not a true alcoholic. If the experts had known me 25 years ago, when I was living on booze with almost no food at all, I think they would have diagnosed me as an alcoholic. In any case, there may be many others just like me who can overcome their craving for alcohol . . . by maintaining the kind of dietary program I maintained."

(*Megavitamin Therapy*, Ruth Adams and Frank Murray, 1982)

After rereading these stories, I did some research, and I found some information that surely goes along with them. I was poking around the medical journal database and found two articles from the journal *Alcohol,* both from the spring/summer of 1999. One had the lively title, "Association between preference for sweets and excessive alcohol intake: a review of animal and human studies." This article stated that in both animal and human studies, the consumption of sweets was linked to the consumption of alcohol. For instance, rats that liked to drink a lot of alcohol were also found to consume sweet drinks—both sugar and saccharine solutions—far beyond what they usually drank when given plain water. The article also stated that alcoholics prefer ultrasweet solutions—that they like drinks that are far sweeter than non-alchoholic folks do.

This article also noted that alcoholics sometimes use sugar to suppress alcohol cravings—that they substitute sugar for alcohol. This interested me, because the folks I know who have been in Alcoholics Anonymous have reported that cookies and cups of heavily sugared coffee are the standard refreshments at AA meetings. It appears that sugar can become a substitute addiction for the sober alcoholic. This, however, can be dangerous—one sober alcoholic in my family turned to sugar instead, only to eventually be diagnosed with type II diabetes.

The second article from *Alcohol* studied the alcohol intake of hamsters when they were on a high-fat diet, and compared it to their alcohol intake when they were on a high-carbohydrate diet. The hamsters (who, according to the article, "avidly consume ethanol [alcohol] solutions"—isn't it weird to think of cute little hamsters as lushes?) were given one of three diets: a control diet of Purina rodent chow, a high-carbohydrate/low-fat diet, or a low-carb/high-fat diet. The hamsters on the Purina chow and on the low-fat/high-carb diet drank similar amounts of alcohol—but the hamsters on the high-fat/low-carb diet drank much less!

This struck me as significant. I wondered if the researchers who found that eating sugar helped alcoholics to stay sober had looked at sugar restriction *along with* restriction of *all* carbohydrates? Or just in the context of the "normal" American diet—the human equivalent of the Purina chow used for the controls?

Well, these two articles whetted my appetite! I had to dig further. I found an article from the Bowles Center for Alcohol Studies that stated that the alcoholic's preference for very sweet tastes was so strong that perhaps it could be used to test for potential alcoholism—the stronger a sweet taste one preferred, the greater the risk of developing alcoholism!

The journal *Nutrition,* in the summer of 1999, stated that alcoholics are usually glucose intolerant. This was echoed by an article in a Japanese journal called *Nippon Rinsho* ("Japanese Clinic"), which stated that glucose intolerance and diabetes are prevalent among alcoholics, whether they have cirrhosis of the liver or not. And I found an article regarding high blood pressure in alcoholics who quit drinking—the article blamed our old enemy hyperinsulinemia.

So, while the exact mechanism is not clear, it appears that alcoholism is yet another carbohydrate intolerance disease, which is not surprising, as alcohol is made from carbohydrates!

NOTE: I am *not* suggesting that a low-carbohydrate diet will automatically fix alcoholism. And I am really, *really* not suggesting that if you are a sober alcoholic, you can start eating a low-carbohydrate diet and then try drinking again. That would be foolish to the point of being suicidal.

It does look hopeful, though, that a low-carbohydrate diet with plenty of protein may well make getting and staying sober easier. And it does begin to appear that alcoholics are at a high risk for switching over to sugar addiction when they quit drinking. I hope I've made it clear that while sugar addiction is likely to be less devastating to your personal life, it can have medical consequences that are nearly as dangerous as those of heavy drinking.

Also very important, is what this tells us about how we're feeding our children is. There is *every* reason to believe that the average American child's diet, with 50 percent of calories coming from pure sugar, and quite a lot of the rest coming from other highly processed, rapidly absorbed carbohydrates, is setting our young people up for alcohol addiction, and perhaps addiction to other drugs, too, as they grow older. Feeding your kids well is always important, but if you have any family history of alcoholism, cutting out the junk in your children's diet is *vital*. It could save them from a lifetime of pain and addiction, and maybe even from prison, or an early death.

Changed Your Mind Yet?

Now, I know some—perhaps most—of you are in severe shock right now. I had the same experience. I used to manage a health food store. Finding out that my body runs better on red meat than it did on brown rice was kind of like having the laws of gravity revoked! For the first month or so, I kept expecting to keel over dead from the fat in my diet! But the weight kept coming off, and I kept feeling better and better—and eventually, I just stopped worrying. And now I have years of good blood work to prove that my diet is healthy!

I've looked at this pretty carefully, and not just for my own health's sake. I took a class, Argumentation and Debate, at Indiana University several years back. (I decided I needed to be more outspoken and opinionated!) When I got to my Scientific Argument assignment, I decided to do low-carbohydrate dieting.

I was required, for the assignment, to argue both sides of the question, so I spent *hours* online, looking through Medline—an online database of medical journal articles. I was looking for some evidence in favor of all the carbohydrate they've been pushing at us—current recommendations are to eat six to eleven servings a *day* of grains, for heaven's sake!

So I searched under everything I could think of: high carbohydrate and heart disease, high carbohydrate and triglycerides, high carbohydrate and cholesterol, high carbohydrate and diabetes. I read abstracts until my brain hurt, and I found *NOTHING* that indicated that a high-carbohydrate diet was good for helping heart disease, cholesterol, triglycerides, etc.

I found several studies that showed that a high-carb diet seemed to correlate with high triglycerides. In particular, fructose (fruit sugar) has been found to raise triglycerides, even in kids. Guess what they sweeten soda pop with these days? High fructose corn syrup. And many parents consider fruit juice—*loaded* with fructose—to be the "healthy" alternative to pop or Kool-Aid, never considering that their children get the sugar equivalent to up to a dozen pieces of fruit in just one big glass of juice.

I found one study where they put the subjects on a low-fat/high-carb diet with restricted calories, and had only half of the group run. Only the ones who ran improved their blood fats—so I guess it wasn't the low-fat/high-carb diet, was it?

I found the studies I mentioned earlier, where children with cancers were put on a very, very low-carbohydrate, high-fat diet. The growth of their cancers slowed or stopped. In animal tests, those animals with cancers actually had the tumors shrink on a very low carb, high-fat diet! Plus, this sort of diet avoided the horrible wasting away that often comes with cancer.

In another study, published in the *Journal of the American Medical Association,* a high-carbohydrate diet used in treating adult onset diabetics was found to raise triglycerides and "bad cholesterol," the VLDL (Very Low Density Lipoprotein, considered the "worst" form of cholesterol), and make their sugar control even worse. A diet high in monounsaturated *fats* seemed to *improve* these things.

So didn't I find *anything* that showed that low-fat/ high-carb worked? Well, sort of. One study in *The Lancet* covered one man, sixty-eight years old, with high cholesterol and a family history of heart disease. They put him on a low-fat/high-carb diet, and medication as well. At the end of a year, they tested him, and he was *worse*. They adjusted his medication, and cut his fat back to 10 percent of calories—surely a very unpleasant diet. At the next testing, they found what they termed a "mild improvement." Whoopee. I don't consider that a ringing endorsement of a low-fat/high-carbohydrate diet.

In fact, it will surprise you to know that despite the highly touted Food Pyramid, the absolute human requirement for carbohydrate is *zero*, but there are fats the body cannot do without. So the question remains: Why are the government and the medical establishment pushing carbohydrate?

CHAPTER SEVEN

So How Do I Do This Diet?

THERE'S MORE than one way to limit carbohydrate in your diet. As you've gathered, I've read a big stack of books and articles on this subject, tried several approaches, and talked to a lot of people about what they've tried. And no one approach seems to be best for everybody.

So what I'd like to do is explain several different approaches you can take to cutting the carbohydrates from your diet and the fat from your body. I want to give you enough information so that you can come up with what works best for *you*. We all know that the hardest thing about losing weight is keeping it off. The reason, of course, is that people "go on a diet"—and then, when they've lost the weight, they go *off* the diet, and go back to eating the same old way that got them in trouble in the first place.

I'm not going to lie to you. To keep the weight off, you're going to have to change the way you eat *forever*. You're *never* going to be able to have cereal for breakfast every morning, and have potatoes with dinner every night, and eat cake every time someone at the office has a birthday, and keep the weight off. The good news is that you're going to feel so great, and be able to eat so much wonderful food, that you'll consider that a very small sacrifice indeed!

Motivation

So, let's talk motivation for a minute. I am painfully aware that most people would quite literally rather die than change the way they eat. In fact, they do it every day. Of all the dangerous things you may be exposed to today—environmental pollutants, drunk drivers, secondhand smoke, etc.—the one most likely to kill you is what's on your dinner plate.

So why don't people change how they eat? Or rather, why don't people *permanently* change how they eat? Huge numbers of people change their eating habits temporarily, but eventually drift back to the same old diet that made them sick in the first place. Why?

Well, many people go into dieting with the idea that this is a temporary thing. As I just mentioned, they're going to go *on* a diet, and then they're going to go *off* the diet. A woman I spoke with who had lost and regained her weight many, many times admitted to me that she always goes on a diet believing that she's going to lose the weight fast-fast-fast—and then she'll be able to go back to eating whatever she wants, whenever she wants, and miraculously not gain the weight back. Of course, she *knows* this is nonsensical, but the dream persists nonetheless.

It is perfectly honorable to decide that you'd rather be fat than limit what you eat. It's *your* body and *your* life, and if eating carbs is more appealing to you than the weight loss and other health benefits to be had by giving them up, that's *your* decision, and no one has the right to question it. There are far more important things in life than being slim. But it's very, very important to understand that certain things are mutually exclusive in this world; as the old saying goes, you can have *anything* you want, but you can't have *everything* you want. You simply have to *choose*. There's no way you can eat a poor diet—lots of sugary, starchy, refined and processed junk—*and* look and feel as good as possible, too. If you spend much time wishing you could have both, you'll make yourself miserable, as this woman was.

What I *really* don't want to hear coming out of your mouth is the word "can't," as in "I can't give up sugar!" or "I can't stop eating bread!" Do you have a couple of big guys in dark glasses who come to your house, hold you down, pinch your nose to force you to open your mouth, and shove the junk down your throat? Didn't think so. You *can*. And if you'll do it for just a few weeks, it will become far, far easier than you can possibly realize right now, due to changes in your biochemistry.

What "can't" really means, of course, is "I don't want to." And depending on your life, your body, your emotions, that may be a valid statement. On the other hand, it may be a cop-out. Because if you were really comfortable with that decision, you wouldn't try to disown the responsibility for it by using the word "can't."

So, the next time you catch yourself using the word "can't" in this way—for instance, "I can't resist the donuts in the break room"—try taking responsibility for that decision instead. Say to yourself—aloud if you possibly can—"Eating donuts is more important to me than my physical and mental health. I would rather eat donuts than lose the next ten pounds. Five minutes of eating donuts is worth three or four hours of feeling lousy, and a five-pound water-weight gain." If you can say these things aloud, and *mean* them, feel comfortable about them, then go ahead and knock yourself out. But don't go giving your power away so that you can lie to yourself about what you're doing.

A very common reason people don't stick with changes in eating habits is *sheer hunger.* This, of course, is the big stumbling block of calorie-controlled diets. Very few people have what it takes to sit around and be hungry for the rest of their lives. Fortunately, this is *not* a problem on a low-carb diet. Once you choose the approach that is right for your body and lifestyle, you need never go hungry to be healthy and maintain your weight loss!

A third challenge to healthy eating is *boredom.* People just get tired of eating the same thing over and over again. We've been indoctrinated by advertising to think of food as entertainment. I was appalled at an advertisement for fruit juice blends that featured a cute kid saying, "You know what happens when you drink the same thing all the time? Your tongue gets kinda bored." I wanted to smack him upside the head and holler, "You spoiled brat! Get down on your *knees* and thank *God* that you have good food to eat and clean water to drink!" Tongue gets kinda bored, indeed!

The purpose of food is nutrition, not entertainment! If you've been using food as a diversion, *do* something! Read a book, surf the Internet, go for a walk, take a class, anything from massage to ballroom dancing to physics. Take up needlework (hard to eat while knitting!); volunteer at your church, the animal shelter, the library, a political campaign. Look, I can't tell you what things you'll enjoy doing. But neither can junk food! Address the real problem. Distracting yourself with cookies or chips never improved anything; it makes you feel a tiny bit better in the short run, and far, far worse in the long run.

That being said, eating *should* be pleasurable and varied. Unfortunately, many people are now what I call "willfully helpless" about food. They don't cook, they don't know *how* to cook, they don't *want* to know how to cook. They're used to getting "variety" in their diet by using highly processed prepared foods—whack-'em-on-the-counter biscuits, Hamburger Helper, stuffing mix, boxed potato dishes, etc.—all of which offer very little in the way of nutrition or satiation, and all of which are simply *loaded* with carbohydrates of the cheapest, most damaging kinds, not to mention all sorts of interesting chemicals. When these things are removed from their diet, they perceive their diet as having little taste excitement (not that *I* would call that stuff exciting!) and grow bored and rebellious. The funny thing is, they were probably eating the same carb-y stuff over and over again. Why wasn't *that* defined as boring? (You know why—for the same reason that an alcoholic doesn't define "whiskey again" as boring!)

I know of two solutions to the boredom problem. The expensive solution is to eat out a lot, exploring local restaurants for fabulous low-carb dishes—lobster one night, Greek lamb kebabs the next, tandoori chicken after that. Hey, if you've got the budget, go for it!

The other solution is to *cook*. That's why I wrote *500 Low-Carb Recipes*—and there are plenty of other good low-carb cookbooks out there, not to mention lots of low-carb recipes in regular cookbooks! Get involved with your food in a *new way*, and you won't have boredom as an excuse anymore.

Then there's *emotion*. It is my observation that people choose their food far more by emotion than by any other method. If it isn't what we grew up on, it's hard to think of it as real food, normal food. Further, it's hard to think of what Mama served us as dangerous, because we know Mama served us that food with love, and that *must* mean it's okay.

Some of this problem of emotional eating is solved on a low-carb diet; for most of us, meat and other low-carb foods are familiar and "friendly." Eating them without a potato or some macaroni on the side is a little odd at first, but the food we *can* eat is reassuringly "normal."

Other people get worried eating low carb, because they've had it drummed into their heads for years and years and *years* that they should eat a "balanced diet"—meaning a diet that includes concentrated carbohydrate foods. Dr. Atkins said that people with unbalanced bodies need an unbalanced diet to balance themselves out, and that makes some sense.

But I think the whole concept of a "balanced diet" is unscientific nonsense. Do you know what the definition of a "balanced diet" is? The sort of diet people have been eating for the past couple of centuries. That's all. No investigation into whether or not that's the optimum diet, or whether all those foods are needed. Just, "Well, people have been eating this stuff for quite a while now, so it must be what's right." Of course, people *haven't* been eating massive quantities of sugar for centuries, nor have they been eating white flour, or Minute Rice, or highly processed cold cereal.

More to the point, *people didn't eat grains at all for the first couple of million years of human existence.* To suggest that these foods are *essential* for human health because we've taken to eating them recently is sheer bunk. Does a tiger need to eat a "balanced diet" that includes grains? No, he needs a balanced diet that includes muscle meats, organ meats, bones, sinew, and connective tissue from a variety of animals. Does a rabbit need to eat a "balanced diet" that includes meat and eggs? No, he needs a balanced diet that includes a wide variety of plant leaves and stems. Why do we assume that the appropriate "balanced diet" for humankind includes foods that were completely unavailable for most of human evolution?

Still, people get panicky, especially when friends and family say, "You're not eating a balanced diet! How can that be healthy?!" My best advice to you is to look at most of those people urging you to eat a balanced diet, and ask yourself if their diet has led to optimal health!

Here's another way emotion can mess you up: You think you *should* crave sugar and junk, even when you don't! After all, you always have. It's part of your self-image, and that kind of thing is hard to let go of. I talked with a woman named Cindy who tried a very low-carb diet, and it worked like a charm. She felt great, lost weight, wasn't hungry, and was *very* surprised to find that she didn't crave sweets. But Cindy thought she *ought* to crave sweets—that's who she *was,* what she was all about. She ate the sweets even though she didn't really *want* them! They didn't even taste very good—but they upset her blood sugar and made her hungry and tired again. A few times of doing this, and Cindy up and quit her diet, and when I spoke to her, she was just starting all over again.

I had some trouble with this self-image thing, too. When I went low carb, I discovered that food still tasted good, I still enjoyed eating, but the huge emotional pull was gone. It wasn't a *passion* anymore. I felt emotionally detached from food for the first time in my life.

On the one hand, this was good; it made eating moderately, to satisfy the needs of my body, much easier. On the other hand, I had always been obsessed with food! If I wasn't obsessed with food anymore, who was I? And where would I find that passion in my life? It was a little scary.

Then I got mad. Why should I have to settle for the "passion" of a physical addiction? What a cheap substitute for real passion! I have a *great* marriage—that sure brings a lot of passion to my life. But I developed two new passions, too:

becoming as good a low-carb cook as I had been a low-fat/high-carb cook, and telling others about how low-carb dieting has changed my life. This book is part of the new passion that entered my life when I abandoned the "passion" of physically craving carbohydrates.

If, indeed, you have been using food addiction as an easy substitute for finding *real* passion, *real* emotion, in your life, it's time to do something else. I can't tell you what to be passionate *about* (although I highly recommend sex!), I just know that food addiction is a cheap and dangerous substitute for real emotion. If you're genuinely scared that giving up carbohydrate addiction will mean the end of intense emotion in your life, I gently suggest that a little counseling may be in order. It's time to find out what you've been hiding from.

Then there's our tendency to use food as a reward. You know, "I've worked so hard all week, I *deserve* a hot fudge sundae (or a deep-dish pizza, or a candy bar, whatever)." Try this sentence on for size: "I've worked so hard all week, I *deserve* to take drugs." Different impact emotionally—but not that big a difference physically, as we've seen. To think of food that will make you profoundly ill as a *reward* is one of the most dangerous things you can do!

But you do deserve rewards! So, right here, right now, think of some other ways you can reward yourself. How about splurging on some low-carb treat that you adore? A whole lobster, perhaps, or an expensive gourmet cheese. My low-carb cyberpal Kathy bought herself a twenty-five-pound sack of macadamia nuts! I think she spent the kids' college fund!

But rewards don't have to be food. How about treating yourself to a pedicure every Friday on the way home from work? You could get a massage; buy yourself some fresh flowers; take a long, hot bath with your favorite scented oil and a trashy novel. Refuse to answer the door if the kids knock! When's the last time you bought a new shade of lipstick? Guys, how about that magazine subscription you've been wanting? Or a full hour on the phone, long distance, talking to an old high school buddy you haven't seen in *way* too long? If you're doing this diet as a couple, I'll bet you can come up with some great rewards you can give each other!

Of course, the big reward for successful dieters is *clothes*! Don't wait until you've reached your goal weight. As soon as your clothes are loose on you, buy at least one new outfit you really, really like. Yes, you're going to shrink out of it, but in the meanwhile, it'll make you happy and keep you on track. Anyway, what better use for the money you're not spending on junk food anymore?

These are the sorts of rewards that won't bite you back. Give this some real thought, and know that you *are* worth it!

Another way that emotion ruins diets is the ol' "I feel unhappy, so I'll cheer myself up by eating X" routine. Most of us think of carbohydrate foods—and sweets in particular—as "the good stuff," a reward. If we're unhappy or hurt, we use these foods for solace. If we're "denied" these foods, we feel hurt and rebellious—like Mommy is punishing us.

But everything is a matter of perspective. We all make decisions from a sense of perceived benefit versus perceived loss. It's all a matter of what's really important to you. People think I have *killer* willpower because I can watch other people eat donuts or chocolate cake without blinking—or, more importantly, joining in. What they don't realize is that I'm not *resisting* those things at all. I genuinely *don't want* them anymore. (They also don't realize that I'm not quite so strong with potato chips!) Why don't I want them anymore? How did a girl who *stole* to support her sugar habit as a child get to this point?

My perceived benefit and perceived loss changed. First of all, now that I've been low carb for so long, most sweet things just don't taste as good as they used to. In fact, most of them taste way, way too sweet—downright nasty! So the perceived benefit of eating the junk food—the taste—has lessened a lot, and the perceived loss of passing it up is almost nothing.

Anyway, if I pass up donuts, and someday I really regret it, guess what? They'll still be making them. Unless the world falls apart, any junk food I pass up today, I can find again tomorrow. (This was a very important realization for me, by the way. As a child, I'd head back to the cookie table at the Girl Scout meeting before I'd finished the cookies I had, because I was afraid they'd all be gone when I wanted more. Guess what? It's thirty years later, and they're *still* making Oreos!)

Then there's the other side of the benefit/loss equation: The benefit and loss of *not* eating carb-y garbage. The loss side of not eating the carbs used to be withdrawal—all the uncomfortable symptoms that came with falling blood sugar. That's certainly not a problem anymore! There's no physical addiction to fight anymore; it's *gone*.

And the *benefit* of not eating the carbs is tremendous! My weight loss? Well, sure. But that's not even most of it.

I feel good. I mean, *really* good. Here I am, forty-five years old, and I have *far* more energy than I did at fifteen! I'm cheerful the *vast* majority of the time! My mind is clearer than it used to be. I wake up bright-eyed and pleasant. I'm not hungry and tired and cranky all the time. Now *there's* a benefit!

You see, on calorie-controlled diets, you eat somewhat like you always have, only *less*. You don't feel much better; in fact, you usually feel *worse*—hungry, irritable, tired, deprived. After all, your blood sugar is dropping, and you're not pushing it back up again! You're on an energy roller coaster, getting shakier by the day.

Not so on your low-carbohydrate diet! You feel better and better, more and more energetic, less and less hungry—while eating food that tastes really great! You're not *depriving* yourself of anything. You're *indulging* yourself in feeling fantastic! And who wants to mess that up?

When my friends tell me that life is too short to "deny" myself sugary junk, I tell them that life is too short to live it feeling lousy all the time! (It's also too short to live it without men flirting with me!)

Okay, end of pep talk! You're ready to decide the best approach to low-carbohydrate dieting for *your* body and *your* lifestyle. Let's go!

Which Approach Is for Me?

First of all, you need to try to figure out just how carbohydrate intolerant you are. The more intolerant you are, the more drastic the change in your diet will need to be. Make sense? So how do you tell?

Well, here's a list of indicators, things that have been linked to carb intolerance. How many of them apply to you?

__ I have had a weight problem since I was quite young.
__ I have bad energy slumps, especially in the late afternoon.
__ I get tired and/or shaky when I get hungry.
__ I'm depressed and irritable for no reason.
__ I binge badly or frequently on carbohydrate foods.
__ I carry most of my weight on my abdomen.
__ I have high blood pressure.
__ I have high triglycerides.
__ I have high cholesterol.
__ I have adult onset diabetes.
__ I have heart disease.
__ I have had a female cancer (breast, cervical, ovarian, uterine).
__ I have had a stroke.
__ I am an alcoholic.
__ I have polycystic ovarian syndrome, or the symptoms of it.
__ Obesity runs in my family.
__ High blood pressure runs in my family.
__ High triglycerides run in my family.
__ High cholesterol runs in my family.
__ Adult onset diabetes runs in my family.
__ Heart disease runs in my family.
__ Female cancers (breast, cervical, ovarian, uterine) run in my family.
__ Stroke runs in my family.
__ Alcoholism runs in my family.
__ Polycystic ovarian syndrome runs in my family.

If the answer is yes to more than two or three of these, you're likely to be pretty intolerant. The more yes answers, the more intolerant you're likely to be. And the more people in your family who have had these problems, the more intolerant you're likely to be. (I had at least *ten* yes answers before I went low carb! Obviously, I haven't changed my family health history, but I don't have those energy slumps and depressed spells anymore!) Keep this in mind when choosing an approach.

The second thing you need to consider when deciding on an approach to cutting carbs is just how much weight you really need to lose to be happy. I've lost forty pounds, and as I said before, that makes me "normal" weight, but does *not* make me skinny. I'd have to become a fair amount more restrictive with my diet to lose another, say, twenty pounds. For instance, I have a couple of light beers or glasses of dry wine every evening. If I gave up alcohol, I'm sure I'd lose more. It's not worth it to me. I'm happy where I am.

So ask yourself: Will I be happy if I go from being a size 20 to a size 14, plus improve my health and energy? (Or from a 14 to a 10. Whatever.) Or will I be happy only if I get down to a size 7? If you want to really get *seriously* thin, you're going to have to be more restrictive—and *stay* more restrictive—than if you just want to reach a healthy, attractive size.

Let us not forget that today's standards for female thinness are *not* normal, either medically or historically. Marilyn Monroe, considered by many the most beautiful woman in the world fifty years ago, was, by all accounts, a size 16. In the 1950s, a size 12 was considered "perfect." Now, that's where "plus sizes" start. Even department-store mannequins have grown smaller and smaller! For that matter, men, if you look at pictures of what Hollywood considered strong and muscular men fifty years ago, they look much more real than today's "buff" hunks. I would encourage you to aim at being healthy and attractive, not at looking like one of Calvin Klein's junkie-models or a ripped bodybuilder. Obsession isn't any healthier than hyperinsulinemia!

(This seems like as good a place as any to put in a word to those of you—you know who you are—who are obsessive about your weight. I'm not certain, but I really don't think that a low-carb diet is suited to becoming unhealthily thin. You're much more likely to reach a normal weight, with none of the health problems that accompany obesity. But I will say this: If you're going to become really nutso about thinness, this is about the healthiest way to do it.)

The third thing you'll need to take into account is whether you're a man or a woman. Unfair as it seems to us ladies, men do lose weight more easily than women do. Often they do just fine with some of the less restrictive approaches, while we women are stuck with the more restrictive approaches. Just biology, I'm afraid. As we'll discuss later, estrogen encourages both fat formation and water retention.

The fourth thing to consider is how active you are. If you're going to work out four or five times a week, or if you have a heavily physical job, you may be able to tolerate a little more carb—but just a *little,* mind you. Remember, even five step aerobics classes a week and a physical job didn't help *me* lose weight when I was loading up on carbs.

Still, exercise does improve carbohydrate tolerance a bit. So, if you're going to work out heavily, you may be able to tolerate one of the less stringent low-carb diets. Your scale, your energy level, and the fit of your clothes will tell the tale.

Two Kinds of Change

Okay, you know you have to change something to lose weight, right? I mean, the one thing we know for sure doesn't work is whatever you've been doing, or you wouldn't be reading this!

Remember that earlier I said you can have *anything* you want, you just can't have *everything* you want? Well, that's very true of low-carbohydrate dieting. On some carb-restricted diets, you never have to give up any favorite food, but you have to control your portions and eat *very* low carb two meals a day. Conversely, with some other plans, you have to give up a fairly wide variety of foods entirely, but you may eat as much as you like, whenever you like.

There are two things—two "vectors"—you can change if you want to lose weight. You can change the *quantity* of what you eat, as on a calorie-controlled diet. Or you can change the *quality* of what you eat—which foods you choose. *The more you're willing to change one, the less you have to change the other.*

For instance, if you were to eat nothing but 200 calories a day of MoonPies, you'd probably lose weight. You'd feel lousy, and destroy your health, and be hungry all the time, but you'd lose weight. That would be a change strictly in quantity. (Well, for me it would be a change in quality, too! But if you've been eating mostly carbs, it wouldn't be much of a change.)

My guess is you don't want to drastically restrict the quantity of what you eat. Most of us have tried that. It hasn't worked very well, and it's made us miserably hungry. We've ended up gaining the weight back. So, just changing quantity isn't for us.

On the far end of the scale, there are many people—I'm one of them—who, as long as they eat very few carbohydrates, can eat pretty much all they want and lose weight. That's a change strictly in *quality*, and it's a lot more successful for most people.

In between, there are some compromises—hybrid diets where you limit quantity some, and also keep a close eye on quality. I'll describe a few of these for you, too.

Be aware, however, that the more of those questions you answered yes to, the more you're going to have to limit your carbs to be successful. These things are *not* carved in stone; I know people who have to stay under ten grams of carbohydrate a day to lose weight, and others who can lose easily on as many as a hundred. (For comparison, the average American eats about three hundred to four hundred grams of carbohydrate a day.) And there are a few folks who will have to count both carbohydrates *and* calories.

So if you were slim throughout your childhood, only started putting on a little weight after the kids came, only have thirty pounds to lose, and your only health problem is borderline-high blood pressure, you're probably not going to have to be as strict as someone who's been heavy since they were eight, has ninety pounds to lose, and has a family history of heart disease and diabetes, along with sky-high cholesterol and really bad energy swings. Make sense?

I'm going to describe several approaches to carbohydrate restriction in your diet. First, I'll tell you about basic low-carb dieting, as popularized by Dr. Robert Atkins of *Dr. Atkins' New Diet Revolution* and Drs. Michael and Mary Dan Eades, authors of *Protein Power*. This is what I do, what works for me. If you answered yes to more than a few of the questions above, this may well be your best bet.

Then I'll explain a couple of diets that are similar to this: the cyclic ketogenic diet and the paleolithic diet. Both of these have useful things to teach us about maximizing our success on a low-carb diet.

Then I'll discuss an approach to low carbing devised by a couple of folks named Goldberg and O'Mara, who call their method the GO-Diet. This approach emphasizes fiber, favors monounsaturated fats over saturated fats, and encourages you to eat cultured milk products, like yogurt and buttermilk.

Next, I'll tell you about an approach that might be termed the "Carb Controlling" approach—a form of carb-restricted diet where you still get to eat concentrated carbs once a day, but use very low carb eating the rest of the day to control your hunger. This approach was invented by Drs. Richard and Rachael Heller, of Mt. Sinai Hospital, and is described in their books *The Carbohydrate Addict's Lifespan Program* and *Healthy for Life*. For reasons I'll get into when I explain this approach, I *hated* this diet! But I know many people for whom it's been a godsend. Who knows? You might be one of them.

Then I'll tell you a little about the best-selling book *The Zone*, by Barry Sears, Ph.D. This book is very technical, and Sears's approach seems best suited to those who have only a few pounds to lose, but some of the concepts are useful to us all.

I'll tell you about a diet I've devised myself, not for me, but for some friends of mine who, for one reason or another, I didn't want to put on a strict low-carb diet. It has been very successful for several of them, and I think you should know about it. It combines some carb restriction, some portion restriction, and a useful concept called "the glycemic index"—don't panic, I'll explain when we get there.

For those of you who prefer the "meal replacement" approach, I'll teach you how to make a highly nutritious, high-protein, low-calorie, sugar-free shake, without spending an arm and a leg.

Finally, I'll go over the basics of low carbing for vegetarians.

Once you understand all these different approaches, and understand the principles involved, you'll be able to customize a program for your body, your lifestyle, and your preferences. And that's a very nice place to be!

CHAPTER EIGHT

Protein Is Key

O N ALL OF THESE DIETS—heck, on any diet—the most important thing you can eat is protein. In fact, that's what the word "protein" means: "first in importance." Your body absolutely has to have a certain amount of protein every day, just to replace the cells that die. And if you get less protein than you need, your metabolism drops. Don't want that!

Further, protein will fill you up and stabilize your blood sugar more than any other kind of food. That's why eating eggs for breakfast will keep you full and energetic till lunchtime, or even beyond, but cereal will leave you hungry by 10:00. (That's why we have coffee breaks, you know—so people who had carbohydrates for breakfast can get another fix and get their blood sugar back up. It really ought to be called a blood sugar break.)

The Opposite of Insulin!

Here's one more reason that protein is your friend. Remember all that stuff I said about insulin? Well, your body makes a hormone that is the *exact opposite* of insulin! While insulin ushers sugar into your fat cells to be stored as fat, and then slams and locks the door, this opposite hormone opens the door and lets the fat back out to be burned for fuel! This opposite hormone is called *glucagon*.

When you eat carbohydrate, your body makes *only* insulin. And if you're carbohydrate intolerant, it makes way too much insulin. But if you eat protein, your body makes only a *little* insulin—and, at the same time, it makes glucagon! All of a sudden, your fat *storage* and fat *burning* hormones are in balance!

So you see, eating enough protein is very, very important.

(By the way, the other thing that makes your body produce glucagon is your old pal *exercise*. You knew it was good for you, right?)

Before I go any further, let me talk a little about protein foods. I learned when I was in the health food industry that a lot of people didn't know what foods had protein in them, and I want to be sure you *do* know. The best protein foods are meat, poultry, fish, eggs, cheese, yogurt (but not milk, which has good protein but quite a lot of carbohydrate, too), and some protein powders.

It is possible to get protein from other foods. For instance, you can get protein from rice and beans, or macaroni and cheese, or peanut butter and bread. However, these foods have a *lot* of carbohydrate in them too—so if you're carbohydrate intolerant, these are *not* good sources of protein for you.

How Much Protein Should I Eat?

Both the Zone and Protein Power diets use some rather complicated formulas for calculating your exact protein requirement. Personally, their formulas didn't work for me. They're supposed to let you calculate your body composition—how much fat tissue versus how much lean tissue—but I got a wildly different result with these formulas (twenty percentage points different!) than I did when I had my body fat professionally tested at the YMCA a month or two later. I attribute this to being built funny. You're supposed to measure your waist at the level of your navel, and your hips at their widest point, and take a ratio. Unfortunately, my navel is not at my waist, but at the level of the widest part of my hips, which threw the calculation way off.

I don't think it's essential to be so precise. So instead of making you do a bunch of math, I'll give you the down-and-dirty formula that's been kicking around the health food industry for years. *Take your ideal, healthy weight* (not *a model-skinny, anorexic weight) in pounds, divide it in half, and that's the number of grams of protein you should get in a day.* So if your healthy weight would be 130 pounds, your minimum protein requirement every day would be 65 grams. This is reasonably close to the government standard of 0.8 grams of protein for every kilogram of active body weight, and a whole lot easier to figure.

Be aware, too, that some researchers feel that your protein intake should be based on your *actual* weight, not your ideal, healthy weight. If you're very heavy, there's some reason to feel you'll need more protein than average, at least to start.

In general, figure that the vast majority of people need at least 60 grams of protein a day, and very few need more than 150 grams a day. If you stay in this range, you should do fine. In fact, I think it's best to eat a bit more than your minimum requirement. As you may recall, your body does indeed need some glucose, and on a low-carb diet you will derive some of that glucose from protein, which means you may need a bit more than the minimum.

Recently some bad things have been said about excess protein. You should know that my *very* conservative nutrition text, where I got that government figure for protein intake, says that it's okay to eat up to *double* your minimum protein requirement for the day. That's a *lot*! So don't worry.

As for the old wheeze about protein being hard on the kidneys, there have been a couple of peer-reviewed medical studies in respected journals recently that lay this to rest pretty effectively. One compared kidney function in people who had eaten a high-protein diet for years to kidney function in longtime vegetarians living on a low-protein diet. *No* difference in kidney function was found. Another specifically studied people on a low-carb diet for weight loss and concluded that "no adverse effects" were found. I did find one medical journal article that suggested that a low-carbohydrate, high-protein diet could cause you to excrete more calcium, possibly encouraging bone loss and leading to kidney stones—in people who ate more than *two to three times* the recommended amounts of protein. That's a ridiculous amount, and yes, you probably shouldn't eat that much—but unless you're really pushing it, you're not likely to.

Not to worry.

So, how much protein is in stuff? Eggs have 6 or 7 grams apiece, and meat has about 7 grams per ounce. So, for instance, a quarter-pound hamburger has about 21 grams. (You'd think it would be 28 grams, but what fast-food joints advertise as Quarter Pounders are weighed *before* cooking, and then shrink. That 7-grams-per-ounce figure is cooked weight.) Cheese also has 7 grams an ounce—an ounce of most cheeses is an inch square cube. So, we're looking at maybe two or three eggs for breakfast, and a 4-ounce serving of meat, fish, or poultry for lunch and dinner as a reasonable *minimum* protein requirement for most of you. (Neat trick: Figure the size of a minimum serving of meat by looking at the size of your palm. Your minimum serving should be about the same size as your palm, both in diameter and in thickness. Your very own built-in gauge!)

On most of these programs you can eat a bit more protein than this if you want (I do)—but you should do your best not to eat *less*. Isn't it nice to be told not to eat less?

Spread It Out

It's best not to eat all your protein at one or two meals. Instead, spread it out in at least three meals a day, and maybe even a couple of snacks. If you eat way too much protein at one shot—say, a 16-ounce steak—there's a tendency for your body to turn it into sugar, and here comes insulin again!

It's a good idea always to eat a substantial portion of your protein at breakfast. This will help you control your blood sugar, your hunger, and your energy all day long. In fact, it makes far more sense to eat your biggest dose of protein in the morning, than in the evening, unless you're going out dancing after dinner. Watching TV and running the dishwasher just don't take that much fuel!

So, protein at every meal, but the biggest dose at breakfast—at *least* 14 grams (two eggs' worth)!

Okay! On to the diets.

CHAPTER NINE

The Basic Low-Carbohydrate Diet

FIRST, THE BASIC Low-Carbohydrate Diet, as exemplified by Atkins and Protein Power. (This is also very close to what was advocated by Dr. Herman Taller in *Calories Don't Count*, and by Dr. Richard MacKarness in *Eat Fat and Grow Slim*, back in the 1950s and 1960s.) This is the type of diet I eat, the diet that works for me, and that I feel best on. For many of you, this will be the diet of choice.

Both of these programs were developed by medical doctors. "Atkins" is short for *Dr. Atkins' New Diet Revolution*. Robert Atkins was originally trained as a cardiologist, but became famous as an advocate of low-carbohydrate dieting back in the 1970s. Doc Atkins was an industry unto himself, writing books and hosting a radio call-in show; he had a line of nutritional supplements; and he ran the Atkins Center in New York City, where he used what he termed "complementary medicine"—the combination of standard medicine with diet, supplementation, and alternative medical disciplines—to treat a wide variety of illnesses. Atkins felt very strongly that unstable blood sugar and hyperinsulinemia (high levels of insulin in the blood) are aggravating factors in a whole host of diseases. Obviously, I agree with him—but should note here that much of the medical industry does not.

Protein Power, on the other hand, was published in 1996 by Drs. Michael and Mary Dan Eades, who run a weight loss clinic in Little Rock, Arkansas. They, too, have had great success treating thousands of people for obesity with a low-carbohydrate diet, and have found that a whole host of other illnesses—from heart disease and high blood pressure to rashes, gastrointestinal reflux, and asthma—clears up when they get people's carbohydrate metabolisms under control.

The Atkins and Protein Power programs are essentially similar, which is why I'm lumping them together. The focus differs some, and the Eadeses' research is more recent, as some information was unavailable when Atkins wrote his book, but living on either diet is pretty much the same. They are examples of what I would call the Basic Low-Carbohydrate Diet.

What Are These Diets Like?

On both of these plans you base your diet on the protein and fat foods—meat, poultry, fish, eggs, some cheese, along with fats and oils, sour cream, mayonnaise, butter. Your carbs are very strictly limited, so much so that a few ample servings of vegetables and a few nuts and seeds will just about use up your carb ration for the day.

As I said, the focus of the two plans is different. The Eadeses' highlight is making certain you consume an adequate amount of protein throughout the day, for the reasons that I explained in the last chapter. So the Eadeses want you to build your diet around the protein foods, with the high-fiber, low-carb veggies and maybe a smidge of low-carb fruit, or a slice or two of low-carbohydrate, high-fiber bread filling in around it.

A Ketogenic Diet

Atkins wants you to eat just about the same way. But the Atkins diet is very specifically designed to be a ketogenic diet. "What the heck is a ketogenic diet?" I hear you cry. A diet designed to make ketones in your body, of course. Well, what the heck are ketones? Ketones are partially burned fat molecules, and are the waste product of fat burning in the absence of carbohydrate.

You see, if you go on a strict low-carb program such as Atkins or Protein Power—the Eadeses mention that their diet will cause ketosis, they just don't focus on it—your body runs out of glucose to use for fuel pretty rapidly. It then burns your *glycogen* (carbohydrate stored in your muscles and liver) for two or three days. Once that's gone, your body has *no choice* but to switch over to *burning fat for fuel*—both the fat in your diet and the fat stored in your body. That fat burning creates ketones as a by-product, and the ketones spill out in your urine and in your breath. You're in ketosis! (Actually, ketones are formed if you burn fat while on a diet WITH carbs, too—but they then burn up, so you don't go into ketosis.)

Ketosis is pretty interesting. First of all, ketosis has a *strong* appetite suppressant effect. You tend to be far, far less hungry than on a carb-containing diet, even less hungry than you might be on the less strict, hybrid carbohydrate-controlled diets. Some people have to *force* themselves to eat to get all their protein. (When was the last time you had to force yourself to eat!?)

Second, Dr. Atkins claimed that fat burning in the absence of carbohydrates is a very inefficient way for your body to produce energy. "Inefficient" sounds bad, until you realize that it means that your body has to burn *more* calories—more *fat* calories— to do *anything* while you are in ketosis than it would on any other kind of diet. (Remember the stuff about Drs. Kekwick and Pawan?) Atkins called this "the metabolic advantage." In short, ketosis lets you crank up your metabolism the way a thin person's body does! This metabolic advantage, combined with the appetite-suppressant effect, means that most people would have a hard time eating enough to gain weight on a ketogenic diet.

(Let me mention here that this metabolic advantage is controversial. Many researchers claim that it doesn't exist; that the only reason people lose weight on a low-carb diet is because they are less hungry, and therefore eat fewer calories. Maybe; I haven't gone into a lab and conducted clinical tests, although the research I've seen is compelling. I'm quite certain that I did *not* eat a low-calorie diet while losing my weight, what with eating meat and eggs and mayonnaise and butter and fried nuts.

Did I somehow eat slightly fewer calories? I suppose it's possible, though instinctively I doubt it. But you know what? *I don't care.* If the only things that a Basic Low-Carbohydrate Diet did for me were to make me less hungry so I automatically ate less and lost weight, while also improving my health, my mood, and my energy level, that seems quite enough for me!)

There's another benefit to ketosis, one that means a very great deal to me. Ketosis seems to affect brain function—it makes many people happy. No kidding! It's very common for people to have a mild sense of euphoria when they're in ketosis, and I have even known of at least one case where a ketogenic diet was prescribed by a psychiatrist to treat chronic depression!

It takes a few days of strict low carbing to go into ketosis. How do you know when it's happening? Personally, I don't think it's that important to know. If you're losing weight and you feel good, that's what counts, right?

But you can find out easily by testing your urine, and many people find it's a good "reinforcer." You can buy ketone-testing strips for about ten bucks at any pharmacy. (If you'd like to have twice as many strips for the same price, you can cut them lengthwise down the middle to make two strips. Make sure your hands are clean and very dry, and don't handle the test square if you can avoid it.)

You simply pass the test strip through your urine stream, wait for fifteen seconds, and then compare the color of the test square to the chart on the jar. If the color changes even a little toward pinky-purple, you're in ketosis. Again, I don't consider testing a big deal, but a lot of people find it motivating. (Another way you may know that you're in ketosis is that ketosis can cause bad breath. The more water you drink, the more ketones will be able to escape in your urine, and the less likely you are to have bad breath. Drinking all that water will dilute your urine, however—and you'll test as being in a less-deep state of ketosis!)

By the way, don't get alarmed at the stuff on the jar about calling physicians and such. Ketone test strips are not made for us low-carb dieters; they are actually manufactured for insulin-dependant (juvenile onset) diabetics, who have to watch for a condition called *ketoacidosis*. Remember I told you that diabetics could lose weight very rapidly because they have no insulin? Well, ketoacidosis is when they're burning fat very fast, *and* their blood sugar is going way up, and their blood is becoming too acidic, as well. If you don't have juvenile onset diabetes, your body will limit your ketone production. If you *do* have juvenile onset diabetes, you've got problems I can't help you with! (But be aware that back before there was artificial insulin, low-carbohydrate diets were about the only way juvenile onset diabetics stayed alive for a while. Read *Dr. Bernstein's Diabetes Solution* for a great doctor's overview of using a low-carb diet to control type I diabetes.)

Ketosis induced by a low-carbohydrate diet, on the other hand, is *not* dangerous, and may actually be beneficial. I believe that its appetite-suppressant effect was designed by nature to help us get through the long periods of famine that were common centuries before—and even after—humankind invented farming. Ketosis has a "muscle-sparing" effect—lets you burn fat without losing any muscle mass, which would have been vital to prehistoric man. If you have a functioning pancreas, you can't go into runaway ketosis like a diabetic would; if you're making more ketones than your body is happy about, it will convert some protein into glucose, release a little insulin, and bring your level of ketones down a bit. So don't sweat it.

Dr. Lubert Stryer, professor of biochemistry at Stanford University, says in the medical-school textbook he wrote that the heart and kidneys prefer ketones over glucose as fuel. So does the brain. I've heard and read that the brain "requires glucose." If that's the case, my brain was dead *years* ago! Actually, I feel wonderfully sharp and clearheaded in ketosis. And ketogenic diets have been used for decades to treat seizures. It's hard to understand how a diet used to treat brain dysfunction could be *bad* for the brain.

I have, once or twice, been in ketosis so deeply that it was a bit uncomfortable; almost speedy. If you feel giddy, or speedy, or can't sleep for a few days, test for ketones. If you're in very deep ketosis, add five or ten grams a day of carbohydrate back to your diet, and the problem should vanish.

One other thing about ketosis that is rarely mentioned, but important to know: Testing positive for ketosis is proof that you're running a fat-based metabolism, rather than a carbohydrate-burning metabolism, but it *doesn't* tell you whether you're burning more fat than you're storing! It is uncommon, but possible, to be in ketosis and not lose an ounce—at which point it's time to start counting calories as well as carbs.

So How Do I "Do" This Kind of Diet?
On both programs, they want you to go through a very strict first phase, to shift your metabolism as quickly as possible from burning glucose—carbs—to burning fat. On Atkins's two-week Induction Plan, you eat all the no-carb food—proteins and fats—you want, but only about two cups of low-carb salad vegetables a day, for a carb intake of about 20 grams a day. This is designed to get you into ketosis quickly.

The Eadeses allow you thirty grams a day, again, with all the no-carb protein and fat foods you wish. They want you to stay at this level until your blood pressure, triglycerides, and cholesterol are normal and stable for at least four weeks—but they don't emphasize getting into ketosis, or testing for it, although most people *will* be in ketosis at this low level of carbohydrate intake.

After the initial ultra–low carbohydrate phase, both diets allow you to add slightly more carbohydrate to your diet—but notice I said "slightly"! The Eadeses allow you to go to Phase II Intervention, which gives you 55 grams of carbohydrate a day. They want you to stay at 55 grams a day until you reach your goal weight.

Atkins, on the other hand, wants you to add carbs back to your diet very cautiously, because he wants you to stay in ketosis, with its appetite-suppressant effect and metabolic advantage. You are to add just 5 grams a day of extra carbohydrate—from 20 grams a day to 25—and stay at that level for a week or so, then creep up another 5 grams, and so on. You are looking for the level of carbohydrate intake where you are in a slight-to-moderate state of ketosis. You stay at that level for your ongoing weight loss, until you reach your goal weight.

On both programs, once you reach goal weight, you again cautiously inch up your carb intake a few grams a day, until you find a level where you neither gain nor lose—*and stay at that level for life.*

Subtract Fiber from Carbohydrates

There is one really significant difference between the two diets, and one smaller difference.

The big difference is this: In *Protein Power,* the Eadeses explain the concept of the *Effective Carbohydrate Count.* They realized that when a total carbohydrate count is given for a food, it includes in it any fiber that the food might contain. You see, fiber is technically a kind of carbohydrate. However, it's a carbohydrate so big that our bodies can't digest it, and we can't absorb it. That's why we can't live on grass like cows do, and why fiber passes through us, keeping our bowels clean.

The Eadeses realized that it makes sense to count *only* the carbohydrate that is "metabolically active"—that is, the carb that's going to push up your blood sugar and release insulin. So they want you to subtract the grams of fiber from the total number of grams of carbohydrate to get the Effective Carbohydrate Count—the amount of carbohydrate that can actually hurt you.

This can give you a *lot* more food in your diet! For instance, the total carb count for broccoli is about four grams for just half a cup. But if you subtract the fiber, you can have a *whole* cup—*twice* as much—for the *same* amount of carb! Green beans have four grams total carbohydrate in half a cup—but one of those grams is fiber, so you can have 25 percent more, for the same cost in carbs. Not too shabby!

Furthermore, there are even a few grain products that will fit into the Basic Low-Carb Diet this way. I occasionally eat fiber crackers—crackers that are just basically bran stuck together. They have 6 grams of carbohydrate per cracker, but 4 grams of that is fiber, leaving a mere two grams of usable carbohydrate per cracker, and they're nice big crackers, too! A couple of these add a nice crunch to a meal of tuna salad. There are other fiber-enriched grain products that will work, too—there are oat bran tortillas on the market that are pretty good, and even some fiber-enriched "lite" breads that can fit into a low-carb diet.

(Here's a plug for *Protein Power:* One of the best reasons for going out and buying this book—it's available in paperback—is that the Eadeses have an extensive table of fruits and vegetables with the fiber grams already subtracted out for you, which is very useful. But it's not too tough to look at a nutrition label or a nutrition counter book, read the number of grams of carbs and the number of grams of fiber, and subtract!)

I feel that this subtracting of grams of fiber from total grams of carbohydrate is the *only* way to go. For that matter, Dr. Atkins recommends this approach to his followers, although it isn't in his book. I recommend that you get in the habit of subtracting fiber grams from carbohydrate grams, no matter what program you choose to follow.

One caution: Nutrition labeling laws vary from country to country, and on imported foods, often the fiber grams are *not* included in the total carbohydrate count. If it seems too good to be true, it probably is.

Caffeine, or No?

The lesser difference is that Dr. Atkins said for you to give up caffeine, while the Eadeses say that there's no reason most people need to do this. It seems that some people react to caffeine with an insulin release, and some people don't. If you find that you're hungry shortly after drinking a caffeinated beverage, you might want to try giving it up. (On the other hand, if that caffeinated beverage was a diet pop, you might want to read the section on diet drinks in Chapter Twenty-one.)

I didn't give up caffeine. But I did find, very rapidly after cutting the carbs out of my diet, that I couldn't tolerate anywhere near as much caffeine as I had. My guess is that the carbohydrates were such a powerful sedative for me that the caffeine I drank just about kept me even. Once I stopped eating the carbs, the caffeine was too much. My heart would race! I still drink a lot of tea, but most of it is half-caf—brewed in a big pot with one regular tea bag, one decaf bag. This seems to work just fine. You could use this approach to coffee, too, or alternate one diet cola with caffeine with one of the decaf kind.

How Do I Suggest You Do This Kind of Diet?

I have to admit that I never went through the very low-carb initial phase both these books recommend. By the time I read Atkins I had been eating low carb and losing weight for at least a week, and I was in ketosis when I tested, so I just didn't bother.

I counted carbs for the first few weeks, until I was pretty clear on which foods I could eat freely, and which I had to be cautious with. I don't count much anymore, haven't in ages. Truth to tell, I don't want to spend my life weighing and measuring and counting things, and I'll bet you don't either. I would recommend that you measure and count for a week or two to start, though, just so you're very clear on exactly how much carb you're getting.

I simply eat my protein, at least three times a day, more for snacks if I want. I avoid all concentrated carbohydrate foods—breads and pasta and cereal and potatoes and sugary stuff—and eat moderately of those that have some low levels of carbs—primarily veggies, cheese, cured meats, dry wine, and some nuts and seeds. If my weight starts to creep up, I cut back on the cheese and the nuts and seeds—and make sure I'm not drinking from a really big wine glass!

This should work just fine for most of you. Focus your meals on the no-, or very low-carb foods—meat, poultry, fish, and eggs. You may have cheese, but both Atkins and the Eadeses feel you shouldn't eat more than a few ounces of cheese a day—cheese is very calorically dense and contains trace amounts of carbohydrate (and processed cheese has more—eat the real thing!). You may have these very low-carb foods broiled, baked, fried, roasted, boiled, however you like—so long as you add no breading, flour, sugary sauces, or the like. Eat these foods freely, as much as you want, whenever you want. If you're hungry, eat! Just eat the stuff with no carbs in it.

You may also have fats freely—butter, oil, mayonnaise, sour cream, and whipping cream. (Sour cream and whipping cream do contain a few carbs, and you do have to count these toward your total.) You may eat the fat that comes with your meat if you like—you can have chicken skin again, *as long as it isn't breaded or covered with sugary barbeque sauce*. The Eadeses feel that you should get more vegetable oils than meat fats; Atkins doesn't care. Either way, it shouldn't make a difference to your weight loss.

To this, add some low-carbohydrate veggies and other low-carb items—a little sugar-free tomato sauce; some cantaloupe or strawberries; a high-fiber cracker or two; "borderline" vegetables like onions and garlic; a tablespoon of sugar-free natural peanut butter; or my favorite, a glass or two of dry wine, or a light beer—to round out your menu. I rarely eat anything that has more than 10 or 15 grams of carbohydrate in a serving.

Oddly enough, although cheese, heavy cream, and sour cream are allowed on a Basic Low-Carb Diet, milk is not, for the most part. We think of milk as a protein food, but it actually has more carb than protein—12 grams of carb and 8 grams of protein in an 8-ounce glass. Atkins disallows yogurt, too, recommending sour cream instead, although, as you'll see in Chapter Eleven, plain yogurt seems not to be as high carb as was once believed. Once you're on maintenance, you may be able to afford a glass of milk a day, if you love it.

Until then, I would *strongly* recommend that you get the majority of your few grams of carbohydrates from vegetables. You *know* that the vitamins and fiber are good for you, but vegetables will also give you *far* more food by volume, and far more flavor and variety, than any other carbs will. Sautéed mushrooms and onions over a steak can go a *long* way toward making up for no baked potato! Tomato sauce, peppers, onions, mushrooms, and wine make "chicken *again*" into Chicken Cacciatore. In fact, mushrooms, onions, garlic, and peppers are my four favorite veggies to cook with, though I have to go easy on the onions and garlic, since they are "borderline" vegetables. Nutritious, though!

On the other hand, if you simply despise vegetables of all kinds, you can still do this diet, by eating mostly protein and fats. You'll just have less variety than other folks. And you might want to take a sugar-free fiber supplement (if you know what I mean) as well as vitamin pills.

Most of you will lose weight easily and have no hunger on the plan I just outlined, but a few of you may have a very stubborn metabolism. If you've eaten mostly meat, eggs, and a few veggies for a week and still aren't losing, it's time to buy a food count book (actually, I recommend that for everyone!) and start counting your carbs. Cut back to between ten and twenty grams a day, and that should do the trick.

There are a very few people for whom even this is not enough. Sad to say, those people may have to count calories in addition to carbs. It's not common, but I've heard of it. The good news here is you should be able to eat *more* calories than you would on a calorie-controlled diet that included carbohydrates. Be aware that there is a point of diminishing return with calorie restriction. It is possible to cut back so far on calories that your metabolism slows down in an attempt to keep you from starving. The most levelheaded suggestion I've read for figuring out how many calories you need is to take your weight and multiply by twelve. That means that for my 145–150 pounds (I know I keep giving a range instead of a single weight; that's because it fluctuates from hour to hour, much less from day to day.), I need in the neighborhood of 1,800 calories. Make sure you get all your protein! Even counting calories, you shouldn't have much problem with hunger or energy loss. A real improvement!

Eat Your Fat!
Don't try to do low carb and low fat! Not only will this not make you lose weight faster, but it's dangerous. Old-time hunters knew that if they ate only very lean game, with no fat

and no plant foods, they would come down with something called "rabbit sickness"—they'd get sick from eating a diet of straight protein. At the very least, 30 percent of your calories must come from fat. I get far more of my calories from fat, and it seems to only do me good. So don't try to speed things up by eating only skinned chicken breasts and dry lettuce. You won't like the results. Anyway, there's some evidence that one of the effects of a low-fat diet is to make your body try to hold on to as much fat as possible—after all, it isn't getting any new fat, so it can't afford to lose the old fat.

Remember, the reason you bought this book is because *low-fat dieting didn't work for you!* Okay?

The Upside

So what are the pros and cons of a Basic Low-Carbohydrate Diet? This is how I choose to live, so there must be some benefits over the less stringent carbohydrate-controlled diets.

Well, first of all, most people will lose faster on this program than on the other diets, especially at first. As I mentioned, I lost ten pounds in the first two and a half weeks. Sure helped me stay on track! Loss does slow after some time, but is still usually more rapid than on the plans that keep more carbs.

Also, there is *no risk of hunger* on this diet. The hybrid diets use insulin control to reduce your hunger a bit, so you can limit your portions without too much pain. But I don't like to limit my portions! (Truth to tell, I eat like a horse. No joke. When I make tuna salad for lunch, I eat a whole can's worth of tuna, with a huge pile of veggies and a few tablespoons of mayonnaise!) Because a ketogenic diet teaches your body to use calories inefficiently, you can eat more calories on this program than you can on the hybrid diets, and still lose. You may eat *as much* as you want, *whenever* you want, so long as you stick to the no-carb foods.

But since this kind of diet also greatly suppresses hunger, most of you won't *want* to eat many more calories! While this is not a calorie-restricted diet, most people do *not* end up eating a lot more calories than they did before, simply because their hunger decreases dramatically. On every other diet I've been on, I had to torture myself by sitting around, feeling hungry, waiting in anticipation for the next meal. *I LOVE NOT BEING HUNGRY!*

Even more, I love the way I *feel* on this program—I feel *far* better on it than I did on the hybrid diets I tried. I'm much more energetic, and my energy level is very consistent. Because my body isn't running on glucose, I don't have any "low blood sugar moments." When I've burned the calories from my last meal, I switch right over to burning stored fat without a hitch—no drop in energy! I'm happier, too.

Also, I'm much clearer mentally, which I like. Maybe best of all, I feel emotionally detached from food. It still tastes *great* when I do eat—but it has no real power over me anymore. It's not the focus of my life. And *that,* my friend, is a real blessing.

This is a *very* big issue for me. I am definitely a severe carbohydrate addict—one serving sets me off, craving more and more. And despite the fact that one of the hybrid diets is a Carb-Controlling program called *The Carbohydrate Addict's Lifespan Program, this* addict feels that the best way to treat her addiction is to avoid the drug altogether.

When I tried the Carb-Controlling approach—described later—after having been on a Basic Low-Carb Diet for a couple of months, it startled me to discover just how drugged and drunk I felt after I ate the carbs that the program required. I decided that for me, a daily dose of my drug of choice was *not* the best way to treat the problem. I prefer, for the most part, to abstain.

The Downside

First and foremost, of course, is that a Basic Low-Carbohydrate Diet requires you to limit the variety of your diet quite severely. This isn't like a calorie-controlled diet, where you can make little bargains, like skipping 300 calories of chicken in favor of 300 calories of chocolate cake. There really is no room for indulging in high-carb foods at all—one handful of M&Ms out of a gumball machine will screw up your weight loss for days. (Well, okay. We all indulge once in a while. We'll talk about that later.)

You have to content yourself with the fact that you may eat as much as you like of the really wonderful foods that are allowed on this diet.

Carbohydrate Withdrawal

Also, some people have a hard time the first week or two on the program. They feel tired and headachy for a few days or even a week or two while their body is making the switch from a glucose-burning metabolism to a fat-burning metabolism. Or sometimes they'll feel great for the first two or three days, and then they "bonk" for a couple of days—feel so tired they can barely stand it. It's then that they're certain that they've made a terrible mistake!

But they haven't! It's really just a kind of withdrawal. Let me explain.

Enzymes are responsible for this. Enzymes are what make all the chemical reactions in your body happen. In fact, the difference between living and dead tissue could arguably be defined as the presence or absence of an organized system of enzymes.

For *years* your body has been making most of the enzymes needed to burn carbohydrate for fuel. Since your body will *always* burn carbohydrate in preference to fat—yet *another* reason eating carbs prevents fat loss—and since most of us have been in the habit of eating some carbohydrate every hour or two, your body gets used to making the enzymes it needs to burn that carbohydrate—*but it stops making the enzymes it needs to burn fat!*

It can take your body a few days to realize that there's been a change in plan and start producing fat-burning enzymes instead of carb-burning enzymes. For a day or two, your body just doesn't know how to make energy! And you bonk.

Take heart! The best treatment is to wait it out—it doesn't last—and to take aspirin, acetaminophen, or ibuprofen if you get a headache Also, many people find that drinking a great deal of water—a gallon a day isn't too much—helps this as well. I try to remember to drink a full glass of water every time I urinate, just on principle. You will lose water VERY quickly on this diet, because your kidneys, free of excess insulin at last, will dump all that extra sodium, and with it your excess water. So keep up with your body by drinking more.

The bottom line is that the vast majority of bodies *will* figure out what's going on. When you come out the other side, your body will have figured out how to burn fat for fuel—and you'll have a limitless supply of energy! After all, even slim people carry around enough fat to get them through several days. You're going to be astounded at just how much new found energy you'll have!

On the other hand, I have known a *few* people who just didn't seem to reach this stage. If you give the Basic Low-Carb Diet a genuine, serious try for, say, three weeks, and still feel kinda foggy and logy, that's a good clue to try one of the hybrid programs. That's why I'm giving you more than one way of eating—because bodies are different!

Potassium Loss?

Another problem that affects some people is a temporary loss of potassium with the water you're losing. This happens because the same insulin reaction that makes your body hold on to sodium makes it eliminate potassium. As a result, you're likely to be a little short of potassium to begin with. Then you lower your insulin levels, lose the excess sodium, and drop a few pounds of water—and with it, even more of your potassium. (Once you've dropped the excess water, things will stabilize again.) If you've gone through the withdrawal phase, gotten your energy back, and then a few days to a week or two later, you lose your energy again and feel kind of achy, weak, or crampy, potassium loss—called hypokalemia—is likely to be your problem. And if this happens to you, get more potassium right away. Your heart needs potassium to run properly! Don't mess around.

Load up on some of the many wonderful low-carb, high-potassium foods. In fact, I recommend *highly* that you do this from the very beginning, whether you have symptoms of potassium loss or not. The recommended allowance of potassium is 900 milligrams per day.

Advertising has given Americans the unfortunate notion that they have to eat bananas to get potassium. Truth to tell, bananas are only so-so in the potassium department—390 milligrams each—and are *loaded* with carbs—*28 grams* in one banana! But a three-and-a-half-ounce pork chop has the same amount of potassium as a banana, and *no* carbs at all! In fact, fresh meat is a pretty good source of potassium in general, and fresh fish is even better.

Best, though, are the low-carb veggies and fruits. Broccoli has 405 milligrams of potassium in a cup, and only four grams of usable carb. Green, leafy vegetables are a *great* source of potassium—except for iceberg lettuce, which is pretty short on nutrients all around. Eat romaine or other leaf lettuces instead. A whole avocado, a *wonderful* low-carb food, has about 8 grams of usable carbohydrate (the little black ones; the big green ones are much higher carb) and a whopping *1,200 milligrams* of potassium! Low-carb fruits like cantaloupe and berries are good, and nuts are a good potassium source, too, especially raw almonds.

Clearly, you can get plenty of potassium on a low-carb diet! But if you're the kind of person who just won't eat vegetables, you'll want to take supplements to be on the safe side. You can take potassium tablets, if you like. They're pretty low dosage; you'll need to take three or four tablets a day. You can also buy some Morton's Lite Salt, which contains potassium, and use it in cooking or at the table. It doesn't taste just like regular salt, but it's not bad, and in things (rather than sprinkled on things) you'd never know the difference.

CAUTION: If you are on blood pressure medication, talk to your pharmacist before taking potassium supplements! There is a class of "potassium sparing" blood pressure drugs, and it is *very important* that you not take potassium supplements if you're on one of these drugs. Don't mess around; call the pharmacy NOW and ask whether or not it's safe to take extra potassium in combination with your blood pressure medication.

Dinner Parties and Cooking for Others

Another big drawback of this diet comes when you're out of control of your food. If you go to a dinner party, and there's nothing to eat but lasagna and garlic bread, it can get pretty rough. I know I can rarely eat much of the parish lunch at my church. Often I just have salad and some olives, and that's it. (I eat breakfast before I go!) Every now and then, too, you'll run across a restaurant where everything is breaded or has a starchy, sugary sauce on it. Chinese restaurants can be like this.

In these situations, you just do the best you can. Pick off the breading (I've been known to eat only the insides of fried ravioli and fried mozzarella at an Italian place. I ended up with a pile of shells, like I'd been eating clams. I've also been known to peel apart the layers of lasagna to eat the cheese and meat, and I've peeled the toppings off of pizza, leaving the crust!), eat the salad, order the best choice on the menu, whatever you can do. It's only one meal. If you're really close friends with the person giving the dinner party, you might ask if they could provide a piece of chicken or a chop or something. You could also volunteer to bring something along.

If you're going into a situation where you have no idea what you'll be served, it's a very good idea to eat before you go, or to carry something you can eat—some of those individually wrapped string cheeses, some nuts, whatever—along with you. I was at lunch at a convention a few years ago, watching everybody else eat vegetarian lasagna, while I was eating soy jerky. Not a gourmet lunch, but it got me through. (I could have had beef jerky if there'd been any; soy jerky was what was at hand. It's actually not bad.)

If you're embarrassed about asking for food exactly the way you want it at a restaurant, or about letting your friends know about your food restrictions before a dinner party, let me ask you this: If you had a deadly allergy, one that would cause you to go into anaphylactic shock and *die* at the mere *taste* of the wrong food, would you hesitate to bring it up to a waiter or a friend? Of course not, and no one would expect you to.

Well, more people die of the consequenses of carbohydrate intolerance—heart disease, stroke, diabetes, cancer—than die of anything else! *Your carbohydrate intolerance is just as deadly as the severest allergy.* It just takes longer, that's all. Take care of yourself.

Of course, you'll want to be polite about this. There's a big difference between, "I can't eat that! What are you going to feed me?" and "I don't want to be a problem, and I know you have a lot to do—but this is a serious health issue for me. And I'm dying to see you! Why don't you let me bring a piece of chicken along, and I'll eat the salad and the veggies with everyone else." Anyone who really likes you will have no problem with this. And if they don't really like you, what do you care what they think?!

Cooking for Your Family

If you're cooking for your family, you'll either have to change your menus or cook separately for yourself. This can take some adjustment but, is far from impossible—you just serve the carbohydrate separately from the protein, on the side, instead of making dishes where the two are combined. For instance, you have a taco salad, while your family eats theirs in a taco shell.

But before you serve your kids the spaghetti and cold cereal and white-flour rolls and desserts you don't eat anymore, I want you to think long and hard about this: The rates of diabetes, heart disease, cancer, and many other carbohydrate intolerance–related diseases are rising *rapidly* in *children.* Your children got half of their genes from *you.* There's *every* reason to suspect that starchy, sugary garbage is no better for them than it is for you. Furthermore, they're still growing and need every nutritional advantage they can get. Just because they like and ask for garbage food is *not* a good reason to let them fill up on unfood that does nothing to help them grow strong and well. After all, if they liked and asked for whiskey or cigarettes, you wouldn't give them *that,* would you? Remember, carbohydrate intolerance has been strongly linked to alcohol and drug problems.

Furthermore, Weston Price, D.D.S., in his landmark work *Nutrition and Physical Degeneration,* demonstrated very clearly that "primitive" people who ate no sugar, white flour, or other refined foods had virtually *no* dental decay or crooked teeth. He documented clearly, in photo after photo after photo, the straight, strong, healthy teeth of the people who ate a native diet, free of the garbage foods of civilization, and the crooked, rotted teeth and ill-formed facial bones of the children after just one generation of eating white bread and sugar. Dental work and orthodontia are expensive, painful, and for the very most part, completely unnecessary *given a healthy diet.* How much money do you want to pay to dentists to avoid having to say "no" to your children?

Also, sugar has been shown to disable the immune system for *hours* after it is eaten. The white blood cells, whose job is to go around and eat any germs that might be in the body, become far less active for four to five hours when sugar is eaten. Sugar also reduces the production of antibodies, which are essential to immunity. If you're being careful to wash your children's hands with antibacterial soap, but letting them have sugar several times a day, you're *way* off track when it comes to preventing disease. Be warned.

End of lecture.

Game Rules for a Basic Low-Carb Diet

1. Eat when you are actually hungry, and then eat enough to satiate your hunger, but not much more.
2. Eat all you wish of fresh meat, poultry, fish, and eggs. (By "fresh meat" I mean meat that has not been processed or flavored in any way.) Eat all you wish of cured meats (ham, bacon, sausages, cold cuts, etc.) only if they have no more than one gram of carbohydrate per serving. Fresh (uncured) meats are nutritionally superior. Use moderate quantities of cheese and cured meats with one or two grams of carb per serving.
3. Use butter, oils, and mayonnaise freely. Sour cream and heavy cream have about one gram of carbohydrate per ounce (two tablespoons)—you can use them freely unless you're not losing weight. DO NOT USE MARGARINE, VEGETABLE SHORTENING, OR ANY OTHER HYDROGENATED OIL.
4. Eat at least two 1-cup servings a day of low-carbohydrate vegetables. These include:

Alfalfa sprouts	Greens
Arugula	(collard, turnip, beet, mustard)
Asparagus	Kale
Bamboo shoots	Kohlrabi
Beans (green, snap, or wax)	Lettuce (all kinds)
Bean sprouts	Mushrooms
Broccoli	Okra
Cabbage	Olives
Cauliflower	Parsley
Celery	Peppers
Chicory	Radishes
Cucumbers	Scallions
Dill pickles	Spinach
(NO sweet pickles)	Summer Squash
Eggplant	(zucchini, crookneck, etc.)
Endive	Turnips
Fennel	Watercress

Onions, garlic, tomatoes, rutabaga, and spaghetti squash all are borderline vegetables and may be eaten in moderation—for example, half a small onion or one or two cloves of garlic at a meal, or half a cup of spaghetti squash. Carrots have a high blood sugar impact, but a few shreds in a salad or slices in a stew are okay. Avoid lima beans, peas, corn, potatoes (white and sweet), and winter squash (acorn, butternut, hubbard).

5. You may substitute half a cup of berries (strawberries, blueberries, raspberries, blackberries) or a two-inch wedge of melon for a serving of vegetables. These are the lowest-carb fruits.

6. Nuts and seeds may be eaten moderately. Stay below half a cup a day if you're having trouble losing weight. Avoid chestnuts—they're high carb. In a can of mixed nuts, the cashews and peanuts are higher carb than the other nuts—cashews are high enough that they should be considered an occasional treat, not a staple. Sunflower and pumpkin seeds, bought in the shell, are terrific munchy food, because having to shell each one slows you down!

7. You may have sugar-free gelatin as desired—and you may top it with real whipped cream, artificially sweetened. (I find that just a little vanilla, no sweetener, is right for me.

8. Beverages may include diet soda; sparkling water (watch out for colorless sodas such as Clearly Canadian—these are loaded with sugar!); sugar-free fruit-flavored drinks such as Crystal Light; tea (black tea, both regular and decaf, green tea, or herb tea); coffee; and, of course, water. About half of dieters find that diet beverages inhibit fat burning, trigger hunger, or both. This problem has been blamed both on aspartame (NutraSweet, Equal) and citric acid, a common ingredient of these beverages. If you are drinking many artificially sweetened beverages and not losing, this may be your problem. Drop them and see if you start losing.

9. Drink plenty of WATER. A gallon a day is not excessive.

10. DO NOT EAT SWEETS (anything with sugar, honey, fruc-

tose, malt syrup, concentrated fruit juice, etc.). Products with trace amounts—so little that it shows up on the nutrition label as 1 gram of carbohydrate or less—are okay in moderation. This would include things like commercial mayonnaise, Worcestershire sauce, etc. Be aware that sugar lurks everywhere!

11. DO NOT EAT GRAIN PRODUCTS (bread, muffins, biscuits, bagels, pasta, cereal, etc.), CHIPS (fried pork rinds are okay—no carbs.), or POTATOES. The exceptions to this rule are a few breads and crackers with so much fiber added that when you subtract it out, the carb count is negligible. How do you know which? Read the label!

12. GET A FOOD COUNT BOOK, one that gives both carbohydrate counts and fiber counts. If it's not on the above list, and doesn't have a nutrition label, look it up. Remember that if you add 5 or 10 grams of carbohydrate from one source, you'll need to cut that number of grams somewhere else. Aim for less than 50 grams of carbohydrate a day, after you subtract out the fiber. Keep close track of your carbohydrates for a few weeks; after that, you should be able to "eyeball" it—but if you plateau, you'd best start counting again!

13. Take a high-potency, full-spectrum multiple vitamin daily. This should be a more-than-one-tablet a day product (you'll probably have to go to a health food store), and should give you a minimum of 1,000 milligrams of calcium and 500 milligrams of magnesium a day. Minerals should be "chelated." It should also include at least 200 micrograms of chromium, preferably in GTF, polynicotinate, or picolinate form. Vanadium is also a beneficial thing to have, if you can find a multi that includes it. Another thing to watch for is a B complex that includes "folate," "choline," and "inositol." These are not the only things your multi should include—it should, of course, have vitamin A, the Bs, C, etc.—but if you look for these things, the rest of what you need should be in there.

Typical Daily Menu for a Basic Low-Carb Diet

BREAKFAST: Two eggs, scrambled in butter, with mushrooms, onions, and green peppers
Pork sausage patty
Coffee, tea, or another carb-free beverage. You many have heavy cream and sweetener in your coffee or tea if desired.

SNACK: Handful of pecans

LUNCH: Tuna salad, with celery, red onion, and mayonnaise, served on a bed of lettuce and avocado slices
Two fiber crackers, with butter if desired
Diet cola, sparkling water, or iced tea with lemon and artificial sweetener, if desired

SNACK: Slice of ham and a slice of cheese, with mustard and mayonnaise in between

DINNER: Steak, basted with olive oil and garlic and broiled, topped with butter and blue cheese blended together, and sautéed mushrooms
Caesar salad, no croutons
Glass of Cabernet or Merlot or other dry wine
Fresh strawberries with real whipped cream (with artificial sweetener and vanilla)

Typical Low-Calorie Daily Menu for a Basic Low-Carb Diet

BREAKFAST: Two eggs, cooked any style, without added fat
One turkey sausage link
1/2 cup sliced fresh strawberries
Coffee, tea, or other carb- and calorie-free beverage

LUNCH: Chicken Caesar salad, made with four ounces grilled skinless chicken breast, three cups romaine lettuce, 1 tablespoon Caesar salad dressing, and 1 tablespoon grated Parmesan cheese

DINNER: Six-ounce sirloin steak, broiled, all visible fat trimmed
1/2 cup sliced mushrooms and 1/2 cup sliced onions, sautéed in 2 teaspoons olive oil
1 cup broccoli, with 1 teaspoon butter and a lemon wedge
1/4 cantaloupe

SNACKS, SPREAD THROUGH DAY: 3 slices deli boiled ham, with 1 tea spoon each Dijonnaise OR 1/2 cup pumpkin seeds in the shell

This menu comes to about 1,200 calories for the day. It contains plenty of protein for the vast majority of people, certainly enough that, combined with the moderate amount of fat it supplies, hunger should not be a problem. It contains *far* more than the recommended five servings a day of fruits and vegetables. And it's low enough in carbs for all but the most severely carbohydrate intolerant. It is a bit low in fiber; but remember that most carb foods—white flour pasta, bagels, etc.—don't offer fiber anyway. You could supplement with psyllium or another fiber supplement, you could add a bowl of flax seed–based cereal, or you could add some more low-carb vegetables for a few more calories. How about some asparagus or an artichoke with your dinner, along with the green beans?

Don't try to make this menu even lower calorie by leaving out the olive oil, the butter, the salad dressing, etc. These are healthy, natural fats, and your body needs them. Also, you shouldn't try to drop even a smidge below 1,200 calories per day. In fact, 1,500–1,800 calories per day is more reasonable, even for people who need to restrict calories. Remember that I don't count my calories at all, and most people won't need to. I just wanted to demonstrate to you how much good, real food you could eat, even if you are one of the unlucky few who need to restrict both carbs and calories.

CHAPTER TEN

Variants of the Basic Low-Carbohydrate Diet

The Cyclic Ketogenic Diet

BOY, ISN'T THAT a mouthful! What's a Cyclic Ketogenic Diet? It's a diet where you deliberately go out of ketosis from time to time by eating carbs.

You see, bodies have an almost endless ability to adapt, and that includes adapting to a ketogenic diet. It seems that you lose the metabolic advantage that you had originally, and it becomes harder to burn fat and go into ketosis, and weight loss can level off. There's speculation that your body becomes better and better at converting protein to glucose, but no one is entirely sure.

Some people feel that the solution to this is the Cyclic Ketogenic Diet. What this means is you eat a very, very low carb diet—that Induction thing I was talking about, maybe twenty to thirty grams of carbohydrate a day, five or six days a week. Then, on the weekend, you eat carbs. Bunches of carbs. *Mostly* carbs! Come Monday, it's back on your very low carb diet again.

This approach was developed by bodybuilders and has been spreading through the weight-lifting community under the names Body Opus and the Anabolic Diet. The point is to burn fat while on the low-carb part of the diet, and then, on the weekends, deliberately use insulin as an anabolic (muscle-building) hormone.

Muscle building?! I can hear you now. After all those bad things I said about insulin, what do I *mean,* muscle building?

Remember I explained that when insulin takes the sugar out of your bloodstream, the first place it takes it to is your muscles? Well, *if* when you produce that insulin you're lifting weights like a *madman,* that's a *good* thing. Gives your muscles lots of energy to grow! But you *have* to be working out *very intensely, right then,* or you just make fat. Furthermore, while aerobic exercise works great on a fat-burning metabolism, anaerobic exercise, like heavy weight lifting, *requires* some carbohydrate.

Even if you're not a bodybuilder, and you're just going for a walk or cleaning the garage on the weekend, it's okay to put on a pound or two of fat—IF (big IF!) you then lose four or five pounds during the week, when you go back into ketosis. Many people find this approach works very well.

This also gives you a vacation from your low-carb diet every week or two. (Many people, especially those who are not bodybuilders, "carb up" only every other weekend. In addition, if you're not exercising *very* strenuously during your carb-up, it's recommended that it last no longer than twelve to twenty-four hours.) That can be something to look forward to.

Or not. I've been at the point for a long time where I have to get quite restrictive to go into ketosis, and my weight has plateaued—I'm not regaining at all, but I don't lose any longer, either. I've considered the Cyclic Ketogenic Diet approach to break the deadlock, and I may do it some day. But believe it or not, I really, really *don't* want to eat those carbs!

First of all, there would be an instant gain of five pounds of water. That comes off very quickly, so it's no big deal, but it's annoying for my clothes to be tight for a few days.

More importantly, I feel *so* much better without the carbs in my diet that I am very reluctant to "carb up" for the weekend, or even one day. I have the awful suspicion I'd feel tired and cranky and sluggish, which is *not* how I want to spend a weekend. If you'd told me before I went low carb that I'd ever *dread* the idea of eating carbs, I would have laughed. Now I can hardly bring myself to eat them when I have an excuse!

Still, I thought you needed to know about the Cyclic Ketogenic Diet. So many people find it an effective strategy that I may just grit my teeth and try it some day. Just remember that during the ketogenic portion, you need to stick to a *super* low-carb diet. And if you find yourself having difficulty stopping the carb-up when it's time, this is *not* the approach for you!

Paleolithic Nutrition

Another fascinating variant on the low-carb diet is the Paleolithic Diet—the idea that we should try to come as close as we can to the diet our caveman ancestors ate, because that's the diet our bodies evolved for. Proponents of the Paleolithic Diet point out that agriculture started only about 10,000 years ago, and that most scientists agree that 10,000 years is nowhere near enough time for evolution to occur—for the human body to become accustomed to eating lots of grains and beans. They also point out that paleoanthropology (the study of very old bones and living sites and such) shows that whenever people went from hunting and gathering—and eating mostly meat, vegetables, nuts, and some fruit in season—to farming, and eating mostly grains, the results were not good. Invariably, the remains of the hunter/gatherers show that they were tall, with strong bones and good teeth, and the farmers' remains show that they were shorter, with weaker bones and rotten teeth.

It's also interesting that an Austrian doctor named Wolfgang Lutz has done research showing clearly that "diseases of civilization"—heart disease and cancer—are in inverse relationship to how long a given population has been eating grains. In other words, the longer a group has been eating grains, the fewer occurances of these diseases, because there have been more generations for evolution to work, weeding out the people who can't tolerate these unnatural foods. I have also seen articles linking grain intake, and especially gluten (a protein found in wheat and rye), to several autoimmune disorders, including Crohn's disease and multiple sclerosis.

If you'd like a full rundown of the Paleolithic Diet, I highly recommend the book *Neanderthin,* by Ray Audette. *Very* interesting. Audette, who cured his own diabetes and rheumatoid arthritis with a Paleolithic Diet, theorizes that obesity, and most of the "diseases of civilization," are immune system reactions to eating food that is not suited to the human body. I know of many people who, having plateaued on a Basic Low-Carb Diet, shifted over to Neanderthin or another Paleo program and started losing again.

Once again, the centerpieces of a Paleolithic Diet are meat and eggs. However, some things that are allowed on your Basic Low-Carb Diet are *not* allowed on a Paleo Diet, because they wouldn't have been available to cavemen. Ray Audette gives a simple guideline: If you couldn't gather it with a sharp stick and a rock, and eat it raw, it's not on the diet.

NOTE: You don't *have* to eat stuff raw, although with many things—like nuts and vegetables—it's a good idea. You're just supposed to avoid anything you *couldn't* eat raw, if you had to. Our recent problems with contaminated meat from poorly run packinghouses have made us think of meat as a "must cook," but, of course, people ate steak tartare and sashimi for centuries. Uncontaminated eggs are also perfectly edible raw. (I am NOT suggesting you eat your eggs raw; salmonella is a real problem with today's factory farming.) You shouldn't eat anything that *has* to be cooked or processed in any way to be edible.

For instance, beans and grains *have* to be cooked, so they're not allowed on a Paleo Diet; nor are the low-carb/high-fiber crackers I eat on my Basic Low-Carb Diet. Soy is a bean and has to be cooked, so tofu, tempeh, and soy sauce are out, and you need to watch for "soy protein" and other soy derivatives on labels. They're very commonly used! (As you may have guessed from this, it's impossible to be a Paleolithic Vegetarian. Cavemen ate meat, no way around it.) Peanuts are a legume, and so are forbidden, along with cashews, although all other nuts are allowed. Potatoes aren't good for you if eaten raw in any quantity, so they're out, as are yams, beets, sweet potatoes, tapioca, etc.

Dairy products are also banned on a Paleo Diet, because cavemen didn't keep herd animals. These are perhaps the hardest for most people to give up. No cream in your coffee—but then, as I'll explain in a moment, you can't have coffee either—sour cream on your fajitas, cheese on your burger, or butter on your veggies. And, of course, sugar, in all its myriad forms—corn syrup, dextrose, lactose, malt syrup, etc.—is OUT. Audette will allow you a *drop or two* of honey in tea, and it seems to me real maple syrup could be used the same way, but who ever uses maple syrup except to slather over their (forbidden) pancakes or waffles? I'd avoid all sugar—even though a Paleo Diet also bans artificial sweeteners. (Don't think they had pink *or* blue packets in the caves, do you?)

Maybe the most brutal, coffee is *not* allowed on a Paleo Diet. Tea, both regular and herbal, is. It's not the caffeine you're avoiding, it's the fact that coffee beans have to be roasted to be edible. If you're a caffeine junkie—I'm one of you!—you'll have to drink tea, hot or iced.

Alcohol is not permitted on a Paleo Diet, nor is vinegar (which means, among other things, making your own mayo and salad dressings with lemon juice only, no vinegar). It is assumed that cavemen didn't know how to ferment things. On the other hand, I've read articles about bears eating berries that had fermented on the bush, and getting swacked—I'd be willing to bet the cavemen made the same discovery. But I'd also bet they didn't make such a discovery every day! I'd say if you were doing a Paleo Diet, you could probably cheat *once in a while* with a glass of wine or hard cider without too much trouble. Beer and liquor, being grain products, would be out of the question. (By the way, Audette recommends "ingesting herbs" if you want to get intoxicated. Far be it from me to criticize, just watch out for the cops!)

Again, the centerpiece of the diet is protein: meat, poultry, fish, seafood, game (if you can get it), nuts and seeds (preferably eaten raw). On a Paleo Diet you may eat any vegetables you can eat raw—so potatoes are out, but carrots, which many Basic Low-Carb Dieters avoid due to sugar content, are allowed. Audette outlaws green beans, since they're legumes, but I know Paleo dieters who eat them, since they can, indeed, be eaten raw.

How close does this come to the original diet of humankind? A multinational, multiuniversity study was published in the *American Journal of Clinical Nutrition* in 2000 that looked at both paleoanthropological evidence and the diets of the few remaining hunter-gatherer societies. The conclusion? Hunter-gatherers got about 55–65 percent of their calories from animal foods, and the rest from vegetables, fruits, and seeds. It specifically referred to the hunter-gatherer diet as "low carbohydrate." So much for the vegetarian myth that mankind is naturally fruitarian.

A Paleo Diet is more liberal about fruit than a Basic Low-Carbohydrate Diet is. After all, the cavemen had access to fruit. However, I have two thoughts about this. First, that cavemen, unless they lived in the tropics, did not have access to fruit year-round. Second, I wonder if they juiced their fruit—Audette allows unprocessed fruit juices on his Neanderthin program, but personally, I'd avoid them. Audette does warn against eating excessive fruit, and especially dried fruit and juice, if you want to lose weight, rather than just improve your health.

Still, you can have a bit more fruit on a Paleo Diet than you can on the Basic Low-Carb Diet; if you're very fond of fruit, this is a plus. I've been known to drop dairy and cashews and sugar-free chocolate for a few weeks in the summer, in exchange for eating extra plums, nectarines, and cherries, which I love. I know a lot of fruit fans; if you're one of them, it might be worth giving up cheese and butter and soy and such to have a couple of fruits a day.

So, your basic Paleo Diet would be meat, poultry, fish, seafood, and eggs; nuts and seeds; veggies and fruit. Tea—regular or herbal—fresh fruit juice (with caution), and water would be your beverages. Since the main point of the diet is *not* carb restriction (although it certainly has that effect), but rather the avoidance of the theorized immune system reaction that proponents claim happens in response to the forbidden modern foods, it's *very important* to read labels even *more* carefully than on the Basic Low-Carb Diet. You have to watch out for soy protein, casein or other milk products, MSG, any artificial additives at all. (As an example, most inexpensive canned tuna includes such additives. Cheap tuna is a staple of my low-carb diet, but it wouldn't do for a Paleo Diet. I'd have to spend the money on expensive spring-water-packed tuna instead.)

I have not spent very much time on a Paleo Diet myself, although I find the concept fascinating. I've done well enough with my Basic Low-Carb Diet that additional restriction is not really alluring.

HOWEVER!

If I were a person with multiple food sensitivities, or who had a great deal of trouble with the other low-carb diet plans, I would try this. Also if I had respiratory problems, since most asthmatics and such should avoid dairy anyway, or if I had an autoimmune disease such as rheumatoid arthritis or lupus or multiple sclerosis, I'd try it. The Paleo Diet has also been very effective for breaking plateaus for many dieters I know, of every low-carb stripe.

If you want to give the Paleo Diet a serious try—if the premise of the diet makes sense to you (as it does to me)—I would recommend that you buy Ray Audette's book. It's very interesting! I had to have it special-ordered by my local big-chain bookstore, and no doubt you could do the same—or you can order it from Amazon.com.

At this writing, there is a Paleo Diet recipe site online, at http://www.paleofood.com/—a useful resource!

CHAPTER ELEVEN

The GO-Diet

S TILL WORRIED ABOUT all that saturated fat? Concerned about the official pronouncements and dietary guidelines? You may be happiest on The GO-Diet. A more recent variant of the Basic Low-Carbohydrate Diet, the GO-Diet was developed by Dr. Karen O'Mara and Jack Goldberg, Ph.D. (Goldberg and O'Mara, GO, get it?)

The GO-Diet is the Basic Low-Carb Diet with a twist: You weight your diet toward monounsaturated fats instead of saturated fats. So while you *can* eat beef, pork, and cheese on the GO-Diet, you're *encouraged* to choose poultry, and especially fish, more often, because of their lower saturated fat content. You are also encouraged to eat plenty of nuts, seeds, olive oil (and olives!), avocados, and other foods high in monounsaturated fats.

Daily carbohydrate count on the GO-Diet is restricted to fifty grams, and furthermore, you are not to eat more than fifteen grams of carb at any one meal (those of you who passed third-grade arithmetic will note that this gives you five free grams to play with during the day). You subtract out fiber grams, just as described in the chapter on the Basic Low-Carb Diet, and you also are encouraged to get your carbohydrates from high-fiber sources: vegetables, low-carb fruits, nuts and seeds, and the like.

Eat Your Yogurt

There is another interesting element to the GO-Diet—they want you to eat one serving a day of cultured milk products: yogurt, buttermilk, or kefir. Goldberg and O'Mara feel quite strongly that these foods improve health, including strengthening the immune system. Certainly, they are good for your intestinal health.

However, these products have usually been excluded from low-carbohydrate diets, on the grounds that they're too high in carbohydrate. After all, a cup of plain yogurt says on the label that it contains a whopping *12 grams* of carbohydrate! Accordingly, most low-carb diets have encouraged us to use sour cream for cooking instead of yogurt, because of the lower carb count. How can Goldberg and O'Mara suggest that you eat a cup a day, and still keep your daily carb count under 50 grams?

Here's what they say: The carb count on those plain yogurt labels (and buttermilk and kefir labels) is inaccurate. They explain that carbohydrate content is figured "by difference." What this means is that, first the calorie count is established, and then the fat and protein content are determined. Once the calories in the fat and the protein are added up, it is assumed that any calories left over are carbohydrate calories. And in the case of plain old milk, that's pretty accurate—there are twelve grams of lactose, or milk sugar, in a cup of plain milk.

However, in these cultured milk products, most of the lactose has already been digested by the friendly bacteria, which give them their characteristic flavor and texture. The bacteria turn the milk sugar into lactic acid, which is why these foods have a tangy taste. (This also means that even folks who are a bit lactose intolerant should be able to eat these cultured milk products.) Goldberg and O'Mara say that because of this, we can count just 4 grams of carbohydrate for each cup of plain yogurt! (Remember that spare 5 grams of carbohydrate we passed just a few paragraphs back? Here's where you get it!)

I was pleased to read this, since I like yogurt a lot. After reading *The GO-Diet,* I added yogurt back to my Basic Low-Carbohydrate Diet, and it's worked out quite well for me. I'm convinced that Goldberg and O'Mara are correct, because I get no nasty blood sugar roller coaster from yogurt, and no rebound hunger an hour later. Indeed, yogurt has become one of my favorite snacks, especially late in the evening.

It is very, very important, however, that you not eat flavored, sweetened grocery store yogurt, unless you are *absolutely* certain it is artificially sweetened! Most yogurt has so much sugar added that it's barely a step up from junk food. And health food store yogurt sweetened with honey or cane juice or fruit juice concentrate is no better. In my experience, even artificially sweetened "light" commercial yogurt has too many carbs.

Personally, I don't buy even plain yogurt very often. I make my own plain yogurt and add flavoring extracts or fruit, and sweetener, myself. This is quite simple—if you can make mud pies, you can make yogurt. Here's how:

Yogurt

- Water
- 1 heaping tablespoon plain yogurt (This can either be commercially made or from your last batch. It's the "starter"—supplies the bacteria that will grow and turn the milk into yogurt.)
- 2 cups instant powdered milk

You'll need a clean 1-quart plastic container with a snap-on lid. Fill it about halfway with water (tap water is fine). Add the tablespoon of starter yogurt, and stir it into the water. Then add the powdered milk and mix well, doing your best to whisk out any lumps. Add more water till the container is full, and stir it one last time. Then cover the container and put it in a warm place for about twelve hours. I usually use an old electric heating pad, set on low, tucked inside a bowl to hold it up around my container, but I've also had good results placing the yogurt container over a hot air heating duct with a pot upside down over it to hold in the warmth. If you have the sort of old-fashioned gas stove with pilot lights, you can put the container over the pilot. Any place that's warm but not hot will do. Don't worry if you let it sit an extra hour or two; it will only get thicker.

Why do I use powdered milk instead of fluid milk? I find it easier. If you use fluid milk, you have to scald it first—bring it just up to the simmering point, and then cool it down again before you add the starter yogurt. That's a lot of time, and an extra pan to wash. I can put a batch of yogurt together in five minutes with the powdered milk, even allowing time to smoosh lumps against the side of the container. Also, powdered milk is cheap, and since it keeps, I can have it on hand all the time.

I actually use a little more powdered milk than is needed to make a quart of milk—it gives the yogurt a thicker, nicer texture. It also probably adds about 1 gram of actual, usable carbohydrate per each cup serving—but it also adds more protein and calcium. (By the way, there are 8 grams of protein in a cup of plain yogurt.) If you want richer yogurt, you can add a few ounces of heavy cream and stir it in before incubating.

You can eat your yogurt plain, of course, or use it in place of sour cream in dips and such—although to get the good of the bacteria, you'll have to use it in recipes where it's not heated. You can also make yogurt cheese, by lining a strainer (put it in a bowl!) with a coffee filter and spooning yogurt into it. Let this drain overnight, and you'll have something that's not too different from cream cheese, although it will have no fat, unless you've added cream to your yogurt. You can flavor your yogurt cheese with onions or garlic or herbs and a little salt.

But the easiest way to eat plain yogurt, to my way of thinking, is to flavor and sweeten it. I like lemon yogurt; tastes just like lemon pudding to me, and the tart flavor of the yogurt blends nicely with the tartness of the lemon flavoring. I just spoon plain yogurt into a bowl, add a capful of lemon extract and some sweetener. I stir it up and yum it down. Easy!

There are lots of other flavors, of course. My husband likes vanilla yogurt a lot—a capful of vanilla extract and sweetener to taste—and my sister has found strawberry extract at her local health food store. Or you might like berry yogurt when berries are in season: put a few berries in a bowl, mash them a bit with a fork, add yogurt and sweetener, and stir. (My husband doesn't mash blueberries, 'cause he likes them whole. He just adds them to vanilla yogurt.) Even little kids like berry yogurt, and there are certainly worse things they could be eating!

I've gone into all this detail about yogurt because of the three cultured milks, yogurt, buttermilk, and kefir, yogurt is the most popular, and, I feel, the easiest to work into the diet. However, if you're fond of buttermilk, there's no reason not to slug down a glass in place of yogurt. Or you could make a batch of genuine buttermilk ranch dressing, although you'd have to *drown* your salad in it to get a cup a day this way. As for kefir, I confess to having no experience with it beyond seeing it in the cooler at the health food store—but I do know that it generally comes sweetened, in various fruit flavors, which once again is useless for our purposes. Still, if you like it, and can find plain kefir, I see no reason why you couldn't add flavoring extract and sweetener to it just as you do with yogurt.

Get Your Fiber!

Not only does the GO-Diet allow you to subtract fiber from your total carb count, but it encourages you to eat a minimum of 25 grams of fiber a day. This can mean not only eating plenty of vegetables, but also eating fiber and/or fiber crackers and crispbreads, and flax seed meal.

A Healthier Low-Carb Diet?

As you can see, the GO-Diet, with its lower saturated fat intake, preference for fish over red meat, and goodly fiber intake is a lot closer to the widely trumpeted federal nutritional goals than many low-carb diets. This certainly makes it less alarming to a lot of people, and may even make it healthier. If you're really nervous about eating lots of cheeseburgers and steaks, and are fond of fish, this may well be the diet for you.

The GO-Diet is also the diet to try if you're one of those folks who gets mixed results from a Basic Low-Carb Diet where blood work is concerned—decreased triglycerides, but increased LDL and total cholesterol. The emphasis on shifting the balance of your fat intake from saturated to monounsaturated fats, combined with carb restriction, should work nicely to get your LDL

and total cholesterol under control, while maintaining the benefits of lower triglycerides and higher HDL.

Let me add that *The GO-Diet* is a fascinating book, and one
of the most intriguing approaches to low-carb dieting I've ever
seen. I highly recommend that you find a copy and take the time
to read it yourself!

Game Rules for the GO-Diet:

1. Eat no more than fifty grams of carbohydrate a day.
2. Eat no more than twelve to fifteen grams of carbohydrate
   per meal.
3. Subtract out fiber grams when counting carbohydrates.
4. Eat three meals a day, and snacks if you like. DO NOT
   SKIP MEALS.
5. Skew your ratio of saturated to monounsaturated fats
   by choosing fish and poultry more often than red meat, by
   choosing lean cuts of red meat over fattier cuts, by trimming visible fat from meats. Add more monounsaturates by
   eating nuts, seeds, olives, and avocados, and by using olive,
   canola, peanut, and avocado oil. Aim for more than half
   your fats coming from monounsaturates.
6. Eat at least one 8-ounce serving per day of cultured milk—
   yogurt, buttermilk, or kefir. With these foods, and with
   these foods only, do not go by the carbohydrate count
   listed on the label. For plain yogurt, kefir, or buttermilk,
   count 4 grams per cup. Do not eat sugar-sweetened yogurt
   or kefir!
7. Aim for at least 25 grams of fiber per day. Do this by eating most of your carbohydrate grams in the form of the
   lowest-carb vegetables and from bran, and also by adding
   ground flax seed—also a good source of healthy fats—and
   psyllium husks to your diet. High-fiber crispbreads are recommended as well. Remember that you still must count the
   nonfiber grams of carbohydrate in these foods.
8. You may have up to half a cup of berries, melon, rhubarb,
   or kiwi fruit per day, or up to half of a small, tart apple or
   pear.

9. DO NOT EAT: Milk, potatoes, sweet potatoes, beets, turnips, rice, corn, peas, legumes (dried beans and peas), pasta, bread, bagels, cookies, cakes, most crackers, pretzels, rice cakes.

Typical Daily Menu for the GO-Diet

BREAKFAST: Two eggs scrambled in half butter, half olive or canola oil, with peppers and onions
OR, if in a hurry, string cheese or a hard boiled egg, plus some nuts and seeds, to eat in the car or on the bus or train
Tea or coffee, no sugar!

LUNCH: Tuna salad with real mayonnaise, celery, and red onion, served on lettuce
High-fiber crispbread
Iced tea, with lemon and artificial sweetener if desired

DINNER: Steak, all visible fat trimmed, topped with onions and mushrooms sauteed in olive oil
Large green tossed salad with olive oil dressing
Steamed broccoli
Fresh strawberries with cream

SNACK: 1 cup plain yogurt with artificial sweetener and your choice of flavoring extract (Makes a great bedtime snack! The tryptophan and calcium in the yogurt are both relaxing.)

CHAPTER TWELVE

The Carbohydrate Addict's Diet

NOW, FOR A DIFFERENT approach entirely!

Drs. Richard and Rachael Heller (Ph.D.s, not M.D.s) are professors at New York's Mt. Sinai Medical School, where they also run a weight loss program. They each discovered separately—before they met and married—that their problems with obesity and ill health were related to the carbohydrate in their diets. Rachael Heller had weighed 200 pounds by the age of twelve, and over 300 pounds by her twenties. She had always struggled with severe cravings for food and an inability to ever feel satisfied. Richard had fallen into poor dietary habits as a result of keeping up with a killer schedule—and came close to a heart attack. They both found that limiting their carbohydrates was an effective way to lose weight, improve their health, and, in Rachael's case, eliminate the incessant cravings for food that had plagued her all her life.

After having treated many people successfully for obesity with this plan, and writing the book *The Carbohydrate Addict's Diet,* they started to receive letters from their patients and their patients' doctors, saying, "My cholesterol is down," "My triglycerides are down," "My blood pressure is down," "I don't need my insulin anymore." They then researched the health effects of limiting blood insulin levels, and wrote *Healthy for Life.* The Healthy for Life plan is similar to the Carbohydrate

Addict's plan, but focuses on the health benefits of low blood insulin levels, rather than focusing specifically on weight loss.

Healthy for Life outlines a plan of progressive options, phasing you into a diet that eventually is substantially the same as The Carbohydrate Addict's plan, or the diet outlined in the more recent *Carbohydrate Addict's Lifespan Program*. Healthy for Life also requires you to choose exercise and stress reducing options. I have often recommended *Healthy for Life* to those whose concerns are primarily health, rather than weight-related. I also recommend it for those whose doctors or families are alarmed at their new approach to eating. Since I wrote the first edition of this book, the Hellers have come out with *The Carbohydrate Addict's Lifespan Program,* which revised the original Carbohydrate Addict's Diet in some meaningful ways. Most particularly, the diet now allows for between-meal snacks. I think this makes the plan more livable for most people. Here's the deal about this newly revised approach to carb restriction:

Remember our two "vectors," quality and quantity? Well, *The Carbohydrate Addict's Lifespan Program* is a hybrid—both qualitative *and* quantitative. The idea is to control your insulin levels—and therefore your hunger and your cravings—enough that you can eat smaller amounts without much unpleasantness—and you know what I mean by unpleasantness!

The Hellers feel that those who have *hyperinsulinemia* (remember, that's a fancy word for carbohydrate intolerance that means "high levels of insulin") can calm down their pancreas's reaction to carbohydrate foods by eating them *only once a day.* You may notice that this is the exact *opposite* of the "eat high-carb/low-fat mini meals" idea that has gotten a lot of press in the past few years. By eating *only* low-carb foods at two of your meals, you give your pancreas a rest and allow it to act more normally when you do eat carbohydrates.

So do you get to eat carbohydrates? *Yes.* The rules of this plan are simple. Two meals a day you eat *only* "Craving Controlling" foods—protein foods, very low-carb vegetables, and fats. You also eat *only* these very low-carb foods if you want a snack.

However, your third meal of the day is your *Reward Meal*.

For your Reward Meal, you *must* eat a "balanced meal." You may eat *whatever you want*, in *whatever amounts you want!* Pretty exciting!

However, the Reward Meal has a *strict* time limit of *exactly* one hour. Now, this time limit isn't just because there's a limit to how much you can eat in an hour, no matter how big a shovel you use. There's a physiological reason behind it.

You see, the Hellers' research also shows that when you eat carbohydrate foods, insulin release happens in two phases. When you start eating, your pancreas releases a dose of insulin almost immediately, to deal with the incoming food—and the size of this dose of insulin is related *not* to how much carbohydrate you're eating right now, but to the level of carbohydrate in *previous meals.* They believe that your body tries to predict from your last few meals how much carb you'll eat in *this* meal. This is why you *must* keep the carb content of your non-Reward meals and snacks *very* low—to trick your body into a smaller insulin release.

The second phase of insulin release happens about seventy-five to ninety minutes after you start eating. Your pancreas checks back to see if you need some more insulin, or if it's already made enough. If you've stopped eating long enough ago that your body has had a chance to notice that you're done, your pancreas will be able to gauge just how much insulin you need. If you're still eating, it tends to get panicky again, dump out a *lot* of insulin, and drive you back into the "eat carbs, get hungry" cycle. This means that it is *VERY IMPORTANT* to stay within the one-hour time limit for the Reward Meal.

NOTE: The most common form of cheating on *The Carbohydrate Addict's Lifespan Program* is extending the hour for the Reward Meal. *DON'T DO IT!* It is *not* an arbitrary limit, remember; it is based on physiology, and going past the hour is a great way to end up hungry and craving again.

Also, you must keep your Reward Meal *balanced.* In the original *Carbohydrate Addict's Diet,* the Hellers stated that the Reward Meal must be "balanced and sensible"—in other words, no dinners of merely Oreos and Mocha Almond Fudge, but they also said to eat whatever you want, in unlimited portions.

However, I got a letter from the Hellers—very kind of them!—stating the great importance of *balancing* the Reward Meal, and they have since made this a *focus* of the *Carbohydrate Addict's Lifespan Program*. They now say that you should have a large salad, and then divide your plate mentally into thirds: one third should be protein, one third vegetables, and one third carbohydrate, whether a potato, or rice, or dessert, a drink, or whatever. (By the way, alcohol may be consumed *only* during your Reward Meal.) If you want to add more carbs, that's okay—*but you must also add more protein and veggies*. If you can't fit down the extra meat and vegetables, you can't have more carbs. (Do I sound like mom? "If you can't finish your meatloaf, you must not be hungry for dessert!" Mom was pretty smart.)

Another change from the original plan is that the Hellers now say that you may skip your very low-carb meals *if you are not hungry*, although you *must* eat them if you feel any hunger, so as not to go overboard on your Reward Meal—and just as importantly, to learn to have a healthy relationship with your body and your food. However, they say you may *never* skip your Reward Meal.

Oh, and please note: It's best to choose which meal is to be your Reward Meal, and, for the most part, stick with it. Most people choose dinner, but I've known a lot of people who have found this approach worked better for them when their Reward Meal was lunch. Choose what fits your lifestyle. If you're feeding a family, it will probably be dinner. You may change which meal is your Reward Meal once in a while for a special event— say, a holiday brunch—but for the most part, you should keep your Reward Meal constant.

Another place where the Hellers' plan varies from most low-carbohydrate diets is that they feel very strongly that anything that tastes sweet will trigger an insulin release—*including artificial sweeteners*. They are *strongly* against the use of diet soda and fruit-flavored drinks such as Crystal Light, and sugarless desserts—except at the Reward Meal—and at the Reward Meal you may have products that contain sugar, if you like. The Hellers also feel you should not chew sugarless gum. They state that the use of artificially sweetened products, except at the Reward Meal, will trigger hunger and cravings, and keep you from losing. As you'll read later on, there is, indeed, a fairly large contingent of low-carb dieters who find that diet soda and Crystal Light–type products interfere with their weight loss, so the Hellers may have a point. However, I should point out that the artificial sweetener/insulin connection is *very* controversial, and the medical journal articles I could find on the subject neither proved nor disproved this theory.

How Fast Will I Lose?

The Basic Low-Carb Diet tends to cause a very fast initial weight loss. I lost ten pounds in the first two and a half weeks, and this is not uncommon. This initial weight loss tends to be mostly water. But even after the water is gone, many people lose fat at a remarkably fast pace on the very low carb plan.

On the other hand, the Hellers feel strongly that you should not lose weight too fast—that you should, in fact, lose no more than 1 percent of your body weight per week. For instance, if you weigh 185–190 pounds, like I did, you should be losing no more than 1 1/2–2 pounds a week.

The Hellers also feel very strongly that you should weigh yourself daily, and then average your weight for the week. They feel that this gives you a far clearer idea of what your body is doing, and prevents obsessing and freaking out if your weekly weigh-in happens to fall on a day when you're holding water from your menstrual cycle or the like—no starving yourself for a weekly weigh-in.

The Upside

So, does this plan sound pretty good so far? It certainly has its advantages!

Obviously, the biggest plus of this Carb Controlling approach is that you don't have to give up any particular food.

If you have a very strong negative, emotional reaction to giving up some particular carbohydrate food—bread or pasta or brownies, whatever—this program is *very* helpful. You can have *anything* you want, you just have to have it within the hour of your Reward Meal. There's a powerful psychological comfort in knowing that you're never more than twenty-three hours away from eating whatever you want!

Also, the Carb Controlling program makes eating out, or with other people, a whole lot easier. And it's a good strategy for family holiday meals. In either case, as long as you stick to your hour time limit, you're fine. (Slow service in restaurants or lingering over courses at dinner parties can be a real problem here.) Even though, for the most part, I am not on this diet, I sometimes use it for one day on holidays as damage control, going back to my usual very low-carb diet the next day.

If you cook for a family, the Carb Controlling approach expands your range of options of what to cook for the family, without forcing you to cook a separate meal for yourself. It can make menu planning easier.

If you're a vegetarian, a Carb Controlling diet increases your range of options greatly. You can still have grains and beans, the usual vegetarian staples, one meal a day. (Although you'd still need to eat a concentrated protein—eggs, cheese, or possibly a soy product—even at your Reward Meal.)

Too, the Hellers do allow for some low-fat products—those that still have a pretty low-carb count—even at low-carb meals, and feel that vegetable oils are preferable to animal fats. They call for large quantities of low-carbohydrate vegetables. Also, the Reward Meal allows for the consumption of the complex carbohydrates the media has been pushing. I'm convinced that for the vast majority of us, fat is not the enemy, and I'm quite certain carbs are not essential, but these aspects make the Carbohydrate Addict's Lifespan Program a lot more comfortable for those of you who are still suffering from severe fat phobia and have not yet made the paradigm shift to low-carb.

The Downside

What are the drawbacks of the Carb Controlling approach? There must be some, because I tried it for about three and a half months and went back to the very low-carb plan I started with. First of all, for my body it wasn't low carb enough. I lost weight on this plan at first, but plateaued pretty quickly. I wasn't happy with the weight I was stuck at!

Also, since I tried the original Carbohydrate Addict's Diet, which allowed no snacks, I was often hungry, especially by the time dinner—my Reward Meal—rolled around. I was often *so* hungry that I started my hour by scarfing down several cookies! This is *not* the best way to begin what's supposed to be a balanced meal. And I found that for me, the hour time limit on the Reward Meal felt like a challenge! I would keep looking at the clock, and then jumping up to grab more food to fit down my throat by the end of the hour. "Gee, fifteen minutes to go! Better go eat some more, in case I'm hungry by bedtime." The fact that the *Carbohydrate Addict's Lifespan Program* does allow snacks, as long as they are of "craving controlling" foods, might alleviate this problem.

However, I think the thing that really made me decide that the Carb Controlling approach was not for me, was how it made me *feel*. As I mentioned earlier, I found that after having been on a very low-carb diet for a while, eating a big dose of carbs all at one go made me feel drunk or drugged. I really missed the energy I had found on the very low-carb plan. I finally gave up the Carb Controlling approach when I fell asleep in front of dinner party company! Embarrassing!

Ccooking also becomes a challenge when tasting the food you're cooking *begins* your allotted hour. I am a person who has always cooked by instinct rather than by recipe, so not being able to taste as I cooked was frustrating. I finally learned to adjust the seasoning right before serving food; tasting it started the clock ticking for my Reward Meal hour.

Another possible problem is that the Carbohydrate Addict's Diet calls for a *lot* of vegetables, two cups at each of your low-carb meals, and *both* a salad and a low-carb cooked vegetable at your Reward Meal. This is part of why the plan works—they depend on all those vegetables to fill you up and lower the calorie count of this hybrid plan. Without them, you might well eat more of the concentrated carbs and higher-calorie protein and fat foods.

Now, I like vegetables just fine—but I'm well aware that *huge* numbers of Americans never touch a vegetable unless it's a potato, or the lettuce and tomato on their burger. If you're one of those who are iffy about greens, the Carbohydrate Addict's Diet is not for you.

So, now you know why I didn't like the Carb Controlling approach to low carbing, even if it does allow you to eat anything once a day! However, I think that the changes made to this diet in the Carbohydrate Addict's Lifespan Program, especially allowing snacks, make the diet a lot more livable.

While I didn't like the Carb Controlling way of eating, I know *many* people for whom these plans have been a godsend, and who have been very successful at losing weight and maintaining weight loss this way. For many of you, this will turn out to be the diet of choice, the one that lets you control your appetite and lose weight permanently. For others, the fit will not be quite right, and you'll do better on a Basic Low-Carb Diet like me, or on another of the hybrid plans I'll be telling you about in later chapters.

Carb Controlling Game Rules

1. For two of your three meals a day, and any snacks, you must eat only protein food with no more than a gram of carb in it, plus very low-carb vegetables, plus fats and very low-carb condiments. If it's not on this list, don't eat it, except at your Reward Meal.

    - All fresh meat, fish, and poultry
    - Many cured meats such as ham, sausage, or bacon (some have sugar, so READ THE LABELS)
    - Many luncheon meats (some have sugar or other fillers, so READ THE LABELS)

- Many canned meats and fish (READ THE LABELS)
- Eggs
- Most cheeses (some have more carbs than others, especially the low-fat kinds, so READ THE LABELS)
- Fats and oils, including all vegetable oils, butter, animal fats, and mayonnaise. Avoid Miracle Whip and similar dressings. Some bottled salad dressings (many are LOADED with sugar, especially the low- and no-fat kinds. READ THE LABELS)
- Sour cream

Lowest-carb veggies include:

Alfalfa sprouts	Greens
Arugula	(collard, turnip, beet, mustard)
Asparagus	Kale
Bamboo shoots	Kohlrabi
Beans (green, snap, or wax)	Lettuce (all kinds)
Bean sprouts	Mushrooms
Cabbage	Okra
Cauliflower	Olives
Celery	Parsley
Chicory	Peppers
Cucumbers	Radishes
Dill pickles	Scallions
(NO sweet pickles)	Spinach
Eggplant	Summer squash
Endive	(zucchini, crookneck, etc.)
Fennel	Turnips
	Watercress

- Onions and tomatoes are borderline—you are allowed up to 2 tablespoons chopped onion and/or one-half of a tomato at a low-carb meal. Although the Hellers don't say so, I would say garlic falls into this category as well—only one clove at a low-carb meal.
- You may have up to 2 ounces (4 tablespoons) a day of milk, cream, or half-and-half in coffee at low-carb meals.

- READ LABELS on condiments—many are loaded with sugar; especially ketchup, barbeque sauce, and relish. Herbs, vinegar, mustard (except honey mustard), salt, pepper, soy sauce, hot sauce, and some horseradishes are generally "safe." You may have *small* quantities of lemon and lime juice.

Beverages:

- Sparkling water (be careful to choose those with
  NO SUGAR OR CORN SYRUP)
- Club soda
- Tea, regular and herbal
- Coffee

All other foods MUST BE SAVED FOR YOUR REWARD MEAL

2. One meal a day will be your Reward Meal. The Reward Meal must last for NO MORE THAN ONE HOUR, by the clock. Less is okay, but if you stop after forty minutes, you can't have another twenty minutes later on. At the Reward Meal, you may eat any food you like. ANY food. However, you must eat roughly equal portions of protein, salad, low-carb cooked vegetables, and carbohydrate foods (starches and sweets).

3. You may skip one of your very low carb meals only if you are truly not hungry. If you're hungry, eat! Those low-carb meals are essential for keeping your hunger and your cravings—and thus your carb consumption—under control. You may not skip your Reward Meal!

4. Alcohol can be consumed only during the Reward Meal.

Typical Daily Menu for a Carb Controlling Diet

BREAKFAST: Cheese omelet, made with two eggs and 1 ounce
of cheddar cheese, cooked in butter if desired
Coffee, tea, or another carb-free beverage, with a
little cream and artificial sweetener, if desired.
Remember, you are limited to 2 ounces of cream or
milk per day in coffee at low-carb meals

LUNCH: Chicken Caesar salad, no croutons
Iced tea, sparkling water, or other carb-free beverage

SNACK: Sliced deli roast beef or turkey, plus celery, peppers,
and cucumbers with ranch dip

DINNER: (Must be completed within one hour!)
Salad of mixed greens, peppers, cucumbers,
scallions, tomatoes, and cauliflower, with Dijon
vinaigrette dressing
Grilled salmon steak
Steamed broccoli with lemon butter
Fettuccini Alfredo
Glass of dry wine
Scoop of ice cream

CHAPTER THIRTEEN

The Zone—Hormonal Magic?

PERHAPS THE DIET book that has made the biggest splash in the past few years is Barry Sears's *The Zone*. Sears, while advocating a diet lower in carbohydrate than the average American diet, and much lower than the low-fat/high-carb diets that people like Pritikin and Ornish advise, still recommends more carbohydrate than the Atkins or Protein Power diets allow—and, of course, correspondingly smaller percentages of fat and protein. He counsels us to construct our meals with a careful proportion of 30 percent protein, 30 percent fat, and 40 percent carbohydrate, commonly referred to as a 30-30-40 ratio. Sears is a pharmacist, and he urges his readers to look at food as a precision drug delivery system, where small meals with that "perfect" ratio of fat/protein/carbohydrate are eaten no more than five hours apart. This is to keep an optimal hormone balance at all times. Supposedly, this should allow the dieter to enter the ultimate state of well-being Sears calls the Zone—a place where thought is clear, energy is high, and hunger is nonexistent. Sears *seriously* disses lower-carb diets, especially ketogenic diets. (Despite this, he is a good friend of Drs. Michael and Mary Dan Eades, of *Protein Power* fame.)

Only one little problem—I tried Sears's plan and, contrary to his assertion, I was hungry a *lot*. In fact, I was hungry *all the time*! And as I mentioned, I *hate* to be hungry. Several other people I know tried it, too, and all of the folks who had been on a basic, very low-carbohydrate diet for weight loss found that they were *very hungry* on the Zone plan, no matter how carefully they constructed their meals to Sears's standard.

On the other hand, on my very low-carb, ketogenic-style diet, my thought is clear, energy high, and hunger nonexistent— the very things Sears promises for the Zone.

The problem, I think, is that Sears formulated his plan while working with serious athletes. *How many serious athletes are profoundly carbohydrate intolerant?* Most of us who have significant carbohydrate intolerance problems have *always* been too fat and tired to concern ourselves with serious sports. So Sears developed his diet around people who have an okay metabolism to begin with. Indeed, the people I know who have done very well with this diet are men who have always been athletic, never had a serious weight problem, and only had a few pounds to lose in the first place.

Another drawback is that the foundation of the Zone is one of those tedious, careful calculations of body fat and lean muscle mass I mentioned, from which you determine your protein requirements—and it allows more protein the more you exercise. So serious athletes get to eat some decent-sized meals, but those of us who are only moderately active get a smidge of cottage cheese or a couple of ounces of chicken. Not *my* idea of a meal! This limitation has led critics to charge, not without reason, that weight loss on the Zone diet occurs largely because of serious caloric restriction, rather than because of any magical formula.

Interestingly, when I e-mailed the Zone Web site, they sent me a letter and some info, including an update to the plan. The update said that if you were hungry after a Zone meal, it had too much carbohydrate, and not enough fat, for your body. Guess what my very low-carb diet has? Much less carbohydrate, much more fat!

Further, since the publication of *The Zone,* Sears has upped his bottom limit on protein, so that even nonexercisers get a little more food. Apparently he got a lot of complaints about hunger!

If you are very athletic, and if you've only gained a little weight since hitting middle age, or since you went on a low-fat, high-carbohydrate diet, the *Zone* just might be for you. If you fall into those categories, and would like to try it, I recommend that you read the book, or its sequel, *Mastering the Zone*, since it's a pretty complex approach, and one that I'm not going to try to describe in detail.

So What's the Point!?

So why did I even bring it up?

Because in *The Zone*, Sears has introduced to the nonscientific community a fascinating and very useful subject: *eicosanoid theory*. Eicosa-*whut?*

Eicosanoid (eye-coe-sa-noid) theory. I'll try to keep it simple.

When I first started low carbing, I joined an online low-carb diet support group, or "list." And on the list, people kept posting messages to the group that said things like: "I didn't have PMS this month. Is this the diet?" "My asthma is better. Is this the diet?" "My rash cleared up. Is this the diet?" "My arthritis doesn't hurt anymore. Is this the diet?" When, a few months later, *The Zone* and *Protein Power* (which also mentions this stuff) came out, it became clear that it *was* the diet—and that we had stumbled onto something *much* bigger than just weight loss.

What the Heck Are Eicosanoids?

The eicosanoids are a group of hormones. They were discovered only recently, in the 1980s, because unlike the hormones we're all familiar with—the estrogen and testosterone and insulin and such—eicosanoids are intracellular. What that means is that they're made, used, and destroyed all within the same cell, all in a split second. Since they never leave the cell, they don't enter the bloodstream, so they don't show up in blood tests, which made them mighty hard to find!

However, now that we've discovered them, we're rapidly learning that they control just about everything in your whole body, so it's important to take at least a glance at them. So here's a very basic explanation.

There are good eicosanoids and bad eicosanoids—this is simplistic; you actually need some of both, but you definitely want to have more of some than of others. They're sometimes called "series one" and "series two" eicosanoids, but "good" and "bad" will do. Here's a short list of things these eicosanoids control:

Good eicosanoids open up your blood vessels, improving circulation and lowering blood pressure.

Bad eicosanoids narrow your blood vessels, lowering circulation and raising blood pressure.

Good eicosanoids strengthen your immune system

Bad eicosanoids weaken your immune system.

Good eicosanoids decrease inflammation and pain.

Bad eicosanoids increase inflammation and pain.

Good eicosanoids increase oxygen flow.

Bad eicosanoids decrease oxygen flow.

Good eicosanoids increase endurance.

Bad eicosanoids decrease endurance.

Good eicosanoids act as a blood thinner, preventing clots.

Bad eicosanoids cause your blood to become sludgy, increasing the risk of clotting.

Good eicosanoids dilate airways, making it easier to breathe.

Bad eicosanoids constrict airways and can even cause asthma.

Good eicosanoids decrease "cellular proliferation"—the uncontrolled growth of cells.

Bad eicosanoids increase cellular proliferation and can lead to cancer.

That's a heck of a list, I'm sure you'll agree! It's clear that we want to have lots of good eicosanoids and only limited amounts of bad eicosanoids.

Certain things that had puzzled medical science for years have been explained by this eicosanoid theory. For instance, we've known for quite a while that aspirin, along with lowering pain and inflammation, also thins blood and prevents colon cancer. No one understood why aspirin did all these things—until we learned that what aspirin does is knock out one group of eicosanoids, called prostaglandins, for about four hours.

For that matter, scientists have puzzled for a while over the "processional effects" of exercise—along with strengthening the heart, exercise can do everything from lowering blood pressure to thinning blood to lessening the pain of arthritis. Turns out, as I'll explain shortly, exercise causes your body to produce good eicosanoids. Mystery solved!

Now, Sears and the Eadeses go into stuff like enzymes named "delta 6 desaturase" and such, but if you're like me, that's a bit too much. So let's cut to the chase. What can you do to skew your eicosanoid balance in your favor?

Guess what? It all comes back to *insulin* and *glucagon*!

You see, it turns out that the most powerful effect on eicosanoid production comes from the balance of insulin, which we've been talking about all along, and the opposite hormone we talked about, glucagon. You remember that insulin is the hormone that stores fat and is produced when we eat carbohydrate, and glucagon is the hormone that releases fat to be burned and is produced when we eat protein or when we exercise.

Apparently, the most important thing you can do to skew your body toward making *more* good eicosanoids and *fewer* bad ones is to keep your insulin levels *low* and your glucagon levels *high*—exactly what a low-carb diet does! This explains why so many nagging little problems clear up on a diet that controls insulin levels. Exercise can only enhance that effect, by increasing your levels of glucagon. (By the way, exercise can make you burn fat at a higher rate even when you're not actually exercising—partly by increasing muscle mass, which needs more fuel than most tissues, but also by teaching your body to create glucagon, which it needs to burn fat. Just another reason to do what you already know you should.)

Of course, since protein causes your body to produce glucagon, another thing you can do to enhance your good eicosanoid production is to make sure you get enough protein—again, if you follow one of these diets, you will almost certainly do that. One of the very real risks of a low-fat/high-carb diet is that by limiting protein intake, and raising blood insulin levels, it almost *guarantees* the formation of the bad eicosanoids. Ready to go low carb yet?

It *is* possible to raise bad eicosanoids by getting *way* too much protein—if you really overdo it, your body will turn some of the excess into carbohydrate—but unless you're really going nuts, eating a dozen eggs a day or a couple of pounds of steak for dinner, I wouldn't sweat it.

Now, there are some things you can avoid, as well, to help this process along. We've talked a fair amount about fat, and how in the context of a low-carbohydrate diet, fat isn't especially fattening or dangerous. However, I'm now going to tell you that not all fats are created equal as far as eicosanoid production goes. Some fats are definitely healthier than others. None of them is as bad for you as sugar—almost *nothing* is as bad for you as sugar!—but some are better than others.

First and foremost, you want to avoid what are called *trans fatty acids*. I won't go into a big explanation, but you need to know that trans fatty acids are found in *partially hydrogenated vegetable oils*. These are liquid vegetable oils that have artificially been made into solid fats—primarily vegetable shortenings like Crisco and margarine. I know that margarine has been touted as superior to butter for your health, but it just ain't so. Butter is a naturally saturated fat; margarine is an artificially saturated fat. Guess which your body is better equipped to deal with?

On any low-carb diet, you'll avoid most sources of hydrogenated fats. They're widely used in the food processing industry in everything from crackers to popcorn to cookies to bread. Since you'll limit or eliminate these foods, depending on which program you're following, your intake of hydrogenated fats will be *sharply* curtailed. Use butter in place of margarine when you fry your eggs, or melted on your vegetables. And if you choose one of the plans that allows some carbs, read the labels on any baked goods you buy and avoid any that list "partially hydrogenated vegetable oil"—and there will be a *lot* of them! (Finding commercial baked goods without partially hydrogenated vegetable oil can be a real challenge. Health food stores should have a few.)

Have you heard that fish is good for you? Sure you have. Well, it's true, and the fatty fishes are even better for you than the low-fat fishes because fish oil has a *very* beneficial effect on eicosanoid production. If you like salmon, mackerel, sardines, tuna, or herring, these are *magnificent* sources of fish oils known as EPAs, which increase good eicosanoid formation.

If you don't like fish—I really only like tuna—you can get EPA capsules at the health food store. They are *highly* recommended for people who have heart disease. Also, because of the eicosanoid effect, they are being recommended more and more for people with arthritis. A friend of mine with rheumatoid arthritis has started taking fish oil capsules and has had a *dramatic* reduction in pain and stiffness.

Another way to get EPAs is to eat flax seed or to take flax seed oil. Flax seeds are a terrific source of this good fat and are *loaded* with fiber to boot. However, whole flax seeds have very tough little coats. If you eat them whole, you'll just pass them through undigested and never get the benefits of the oil or the fiber. You'll want to either buy flax seed meal—available in health food stores—or grind your own flax seeds using a food processor, a blender, or—best of all—an electric coffee grinder you keep just for this purpose. Since flax oil goes rancid pretty quickly once the seeds are ground, I like to grind my own flax seed meal. Flax seed meal and flax seed oil should *always* be kept refrigerated in air-tight containers.

You could also eat low-carb flax seed cereal, of which there are a few on the market. These tend to be quite good, and a bowl of high-protein, low-carb hot cereal for breakfast or a late-night snack is a very agreeable way to get your flax seed. I'm particularly fond of one called Cream of Flax; I think the taste and the texture are excellent.

There are also fatty acids called GLAs, which can improve good eicosanoid production. GLAs are found at high levels in breastmilk, although not in most common foods. There's a trace of GLA in oatmeal, but not enough to make it worth the carbs, if you ask me. You can, however, buy supplements of GLA-containing oils—either evening primrose oil or borage oil. GLA supplements have a potent enough effect that they are used by many nutritionists to treat PMS, eczema, allergies, arthritis, immune disorders, high blood pressure and cholesterol, alcoholism, MS, lupus, scleroderma, and other diseases. *This* is the power of controlling eicosanoids.

Also, do you remember back in Chapter Six when I mentioned that a few people would have trouble with something called arachidonic acid?

I said that most people would be able to eat beef and eggs with no problem, but that some people were sensitive to a chemical called arachidonic acid and would need to limit those foods or they'd be at risk for high cholesterol. It now appears that perhaps the reason some people have a bad blood cholesterol reaction to red meat and eggs has to do with their sensitivity to arachidonic acid, rather than the actual fat and cholesterol in those foods. Are you sensitive? Possible symptoms of arachidonic acid (AA) sensitivity include:

Chronic fatigue
Poor or restless sleep
Difficulty waking up; grogginess
Brittle hair and nails
Constipation
Dry, flaky skin
Proneness to rashes

As I mentioned earlier, if you should get your cholesterol checked and find that, unlike most people's, it's gone *up* instead of *down* on a low-carb diet, the problem may be sensitivity to arachidonic acid.

If you think this is your problem, you'll want to eat more poultry and fish and less red meat. You can also buy lean meats and cut off all visible fat. Again, it's those low-protein and—fat/high-carbohydrate grains they feed meat animals that make them high in cholesterol and cause them to produce bad eicosanoids, too—and increases their AA levels. Game, by the way, not having been fed all that grain, is low in AA. Another thing you can do is to marinate steaks and roasts in red wine and olive oil, with maybe a little garlic, for a few hours before cooking. The alcohol dissolves some of the AA, which is replaced by the healthier olive oil. Tastes great, too.

If you suspect you are AA sensitive, you'll want to go back to throwing away some egg yolks; they're high in AA. You could use egg substitutes, if you prefer, but they always tasted really fake to me, and I don't trust the chemicals in them. It seems simpler to just throw away every other yolk when you're making scrambled eggs.

HOWEVER! Remember that the *most* important thing you can do to regulate eicosanoid production is *limiting insulin*. For most people, just eliminating high-carb foods from the diet will cause a *big* improvement in eicosanoid balance. The vast majority of you will *not* need to get radical about cutting out meat fat or throwing away egg yolks. Again, I usually eat three eggs a day and plenty of red meat, and my cholesterol couldn't be better. Pay attention to your own body.

In *The Zone*, Sears wants people to treat food as a drug, painstakingly administered to get one into the optimal eicosanoid balance. He disapproves of using fish oil and GLA supplements to enhance eicosanoid balance—in fact, he states that it is best not to use nutritional supplements at all.

But how many people want to live that way? I don't want to eat that carefully, and I bet you don't either. I'd rather improve my eicosanoid balance *radically* by limiting my insulin levels and exercising, and then take EPAs and GLAs to adjust it as needed. On any of the programs outlined in this book, your eicosanoid balance—and your health—should improve dramatically!

CHAPTER FOURTEEN

The Careful Carb Diet

T HE GENESIS OF the Careful Carb Diet was a nutritional discussion with some e-mail pals. The discussion turned to nutrition, and I mentioned that fructose—fruit sugar—has been proven to raise triglycerides. One member of the group, Rob Douvres, posted back:

> THIS IS NOT WHAT I WANT TO HEAR WHEN I'M FORCE FEEDING MYSELF FRUIT EVERY DAY AND MY TRIGLYCERIDES ARE OVER 1,200. OVER 1,200?

Thus began a very long e-mail discussion!

It turned out that Rob's health was *very* fragile. After seven years—*seven years!*—of trying to improve his health by eating a low-fat diet with lots of fruit—six to eight pieces a day—low-fat cereal, skim milk, pasta and grains, only lean proteins, no eggs or cheese, and very little red meat, Rob's condition remained unimproved. He had total cholesterol of 425, triglycerides at a whopping 1,260 (anything over *200* is bad, and it's beginning to appear that it's best to have them below 100). He'd fought a weight problem since youth, and his blood pressure had been high since his teens. Furthermore, at the age of forty-four, Rob had already had two strokes from severe blood sugar drops! It was clear that Rob was as carbohydrate intolerant as they come.

However, I couldn't put Rob on a strict low-carb diet because he had terrible kidneys. Rob had only 20 percent of normal kidney function, and between this and the high blood pressure, he took three different diuretics (water pills) daily. While it is untrue that a high-protein diet damages healthy kidneys (Rob's damage came from a long habit of heavy drinking, which he had quit years before), for someone with Rob's kidney troubles, an unlimited protein ketogenic diet would have been risky.

But we *had* to get Rob's insulin levels down! So I created a diet just for Rob. And we didn't have to wait long to see if we were on the right track. Because of his serious health problems, Rob gets blood work done every three months—and he was scheduled to have blood drawn just two weeks after he started on the program I wrote for him. His blood work stats hadn't changed much in years, so we knew that any improvement—or, God forbid, deterioration—would be due to the new diet.

And it worked! Here's an e-mail Rob posted to our online discussion group after *one week* on what I'm now calling the Careful Carb Diet:

MY BLOOD PRESSURE HAS BEEN ABOUT 140/100 FOR YEARS AND NOTHING WOULD WORK TO REPAIR IT. I'VE BEEN ON BP PILLS ON/OFF SINCE 18. YESTERDAY AT THE DRUGSTORE, AFTER ONE WEEK ON "DANA'S MIRACLE CURE DIET FOR LIFE," I WEIGHED IN WITH A 10 LB. LOSS AND MY BP WAS 121/83!!!!!!!! MY WEIGHT WAS DOWN TO BEGIN WITH, BUT WAS STUCK FOR 6 MONTHS. I COULD NEVER GET UNDER THAT WEIGHT ON THE "NO-FAT DIET." MY LOW BLOOD SUGAR PROBLEMS ARE GONE, THE VERTIGO IS GONE, I NEVER HAVE HUNGER PAINS, AND I CHEAT A LITTLE MOST EVENINGS AND DON'T TELL DANA!! IT'S HARD TO EAT ALL THE "EVIL" FOOD BUT IT SURE IS FUN!! MY BLOOD REPORT WILL TELL ME MORE. I'M MORE INTERESTED IN LOWERING CHOLESTEROL/ TRIGLYCERIDES THAN LOSING WEIGHT.

Another wonderful thing that happened to Rob was that his legs stopped aching. You see, Rob retained so much water, despite all the diuretics, that it made his legs ache terribly every night. He would have to take both prescription painkillers and prescription sleeping pills to get any shut-eye at all. Yet in less than two weeks, I received this post:

I'M UP AND AT 'EM SINCE 8:30. I WENT TO BED AT 1AM AND WAS ASLEEP IN MINUTES WITH AN OVER THE COUNTER, NONADDICTIVE SLEEPING PILL AND NO XANAX. I'M JUST SPEECHLESS. YOU HAVE NO IDEA HOW WONDERFUL IT IS TO SIMPLY GO TO SLEEP.

Still, the big test would be the blood work.

Just sixteen days after Rob started on the Careful Carb Diet, the verdict was in. His cholesterol went down 90 points, his triglycerides dropped more than *600 points*. His blood pressure was normal, even a little low. His oh-so-important cholesterol/HDL ratio had improved by 7 points. Maybe best of all, his creatinine—a measure of kidney function—had improved for the first time in five years. And fifteen pounds were gone, with no hunger. All of this by *adding* eggs and meat and cheese *back* to Rob's diet—but dramatically *lessening* the quantity and *improving* the quality of the carbohydrates he was eating.

Since then, Rob has gotten blood work again, and all of his stats continue to improve. He's not completely well yet, and due to his kidney damage, he will always have health problems. But he feels better than he has in *years,* and his weight has stabilized around his high school weight. Rob continues to rave about how much better he feels, how unhungry he is, and how much energy he has. And he tells everyone who will listen about how a low-fat diet turned out to be part of his problem, and a low-carb diet, the solution.

Since then, I have recommended a similar program for a number of people, largely those who cared about health first, weight loss second, since weight loss tends to be less dramatic on the Careful Carb Diet. The results have been excellent!

My friend Charlotte, who had been plagued by severe fatigue and horrible mood swings, contacted me four days after she began the Careful Carb program—using one of the shakes I describe in the next section as one of her carbs everyday—to say that she hadn't felt so good since she was a teenager. Charlotte runs a beauty school and needs all the energy she can get, and now she has it! She's lost a dress size, and her moods have leveled out. Further, her blood pressure, which had always been high even with medication, has come down, and her doctor is quite pleased. She's very happy!

My husband's friend called me, begging me to talk to his mother, who had multiple health problems, including high blood pressure, severe asthma, dangerous obesity, and some very ugly mood swings. After a few weeks on the Careful Carb Diet, she told me that she was down a size for dresses and underwear (she's heavy enough that she can't weigh herself on her bathroom scale). Her energy and moods were far better, she was healing faster than she could ever remember, her blood pressure was improving, and her asthma had abated to the point where she'd been able to drastically reduce her use of corticosteroids.

(Here's the cautionary tale: When I talked to this woman several weeks after that, she told me she'd grown lax about following the diet—and her asthma and blood pressure were troubling her badly again. This stuff works only if you continue to do it!)

So, what is the Careful Carb Diet? Well, it's a hybrid diet—one that allows some carbs. Further, unlike the Carb Controlling approach, it allows you to spread your carbs throughout the day. *However*—those carbs must be chosen from a limited list of what I call *low-impact carbohydrates*.

What's a Low-Impact Carbohydrate?

A low-impact carbohydrate is a carbohydrate that has a relatively small effect on blood sugar levels. In general, the faster and higher blood sugar goes up, the faster and harder it comes down. Therefore, low-impact carbs are less likely to cause a severe insulin release, with all its bad effects. The official medical name for these carbs is "low glycemic index" carbs, but that's a little technical, don't you think?

How do we know which carbs are low impact? Since the concept of the glycemic index originated, many tests have been done—and what tests! Medical researchers feed a large group of subjects, some with diabetes and some without, a carefully measured portion of a particular carbohydrate food. These portions are calculated to be worth exactly 50 grams of carbohydrate, not just a certain number of grams of the food. (In other words, a subject would eat a *lot* more cucumbers than they would spaghetti.)

Once they've eaten the food, their blood is drawn, and their blood sugar measured, every half-hour for six hours. All of the blood tests of all the different subjects are averaged so they can get a clear idea of how the *average* person will react to these foods. Then the foods are rated against an "index food"—usually glucose but sometimes commercial white bread. Whichever index food the researchers choose is rated a 100. All the other foods are assigned a number higher or lower that indicates that food's relative impact on blood sugar.

(Good to know: When glucose is used as the reference food, white bread is about a 70, and when white bread is used as a reference food, glucose ends up being something like 130 or 140. If you're consulting a chart of glycemic indices, it's important to know which reference food they're using, or you won't fully understand the numbers.)

I've looked over some fairly extensive tables of these results, and I find them fascinating! There are some real surprises.

For instance, for the past twenty years or so, we've had "complex carbohydrates"—starches—pushed at us. We've been told that they're not hard on the body the way sugar is, because, after all, they break down more slowly and give us "sustained energy."

Piffle! Table sugar, poisonous as it is (and I'm convinced it's as deadly a drug as heroin or cocaine—seems like those white, crystalline powders from plants are just a bad idea, period!), has a much lower impact on blood sugar than does the dieter's darling, the baked potato. In fact, potatoes come in at a whopping 98, just two points lower than glucose! Rice cakes—you know, those nasty, flavorless Styrofoam-like things you've been eating all these years because you thought they were good for you—are a 77. No wonder they never filled you up! And almost all cold cereals are sky-high, even the ones that don't have a ton of sugar added. (Do you know what food has perhaps the highest glycemic index of any tested, with a heavier-duty blood sugar impact than pure glucose? Tofutti, the tofu "ice cream" sold in health food stores. On the glucose scale, it's a 115, while real, full-fat ice cream is only a 61.)

So, complex carbohydrates are *not* necessarily easier on your body than sugar is.

Science has not yet determined all the factors that affect the impact of carbohydrates. But we do know a few things. Carbohydrates that contain a lot of fiber tend to have a lower impact than those that have the fiber taken out. Apparently, the fiber acts a little like a sponge, slowing the absorption of the carbohydrate a bit. This probably explains why whole or very coarsely ground grains have a milder impact than those that are finely ground—in fact, the less processed the grain, the better. We also know that eating a food with a fairly high impact with a lot of low-impact foods, especially protein and fat, will lessen its impact.

But there are some things we can't explain. For instance, whole wheat pita bread has a lower impact on blood sugar than regular whole wheat bread. Why? You got me! It just does, that's all. Barley and rye have a far lower impact than rice or wheat; again, why that should be so is anybody's guess. But the nice thing is that we don't have to totally understand this principle to put it to work!

Here's the Plan

Here's how the Careful Carb Diet works: Just like the other diets, you build your plan around protein. You should aim at getting right around your daily protein requirement, or just a little higher, every day. Don't drop below your protein requirement, but unlike the Basic Low-Carb Diet, it is recommended that you don't exceed this amount by a whole lot, either. Your protein should be divided up between at least three meals a day—more, if you like—but you should always get at least 14 grams of protein for breakfast, and 21 isn't excessive. (Why not 15 to 20 grams? Because an egg or an ounce of meat has about 7 grams of protein, of course! So we're talking two or three eggs, or two or three ounces of meat or cheese, or any combination thereof.)

Once you've had your breakfast, don't eat again until you're hungry! And only eat when you're actually *hungry*, rather than because it's "time to eat," or you're bored, or there's food in front of you. But when you're hungry, eat! Just make sure that when you do, *you include some of your protein ration for the day each time.*

You may have all the low-carb vegetables you like, and moderate quantities of "borderline" vegetables—see the list in the Game Rules.

Fat intake should be moderate, but not restricted. What do I mean by that? I mean that it's okay to eat the fats that come as part of protein foods—meat and eggs and chicken skin—but that you should use separated fats—oil, butter, mayonnaise, sour cream, heavy cream—in modest quantities. A tablespoon of oil on your salad, a teaspoon or two of butter to fry your eggs, a dollop of mayo in your tuna fish, or a splash of cream in your coffee, fine. Just don't go nuts. It's also probably best to choose leaner meats rather than fattier ones.

It's also wise to use cheese and nuts in moderation. This is, again, a hybrid diet—some carb control, some calorie control—and cheese and nuts are *very* calorically dense. If you're like me, it's easy to go through 500 calories' worth of nuts without even thinking about it! It's a good idea to buy your nuts and seeds in the shell. If you have to crack each one to eat it, it's hard to go too far overboard.

You may, if you like, choose reduced-fat products *IF*—and this is a big if—they aren't loaded with sugars, starches, and chemicals. For example, reduced-fat cheeses will probably be okay, but most low-fat salad dressings most definitely are not. Remember that list of ingredients in the fat-free ranch dressing! Those fat-free salad dressings are mostly sugar.

On the other hand, remember that your body needs healthy fats! Don't be afraid to use a little olive oil, avocados, fatty fish. Believe it or not, there are fats that are essential to fat burning! Don't make this into a low-fat diet. It's a *moderate*-fat diet.

Now, for those carbs. On the Careful Carb Diet, you may have one to three *small* servings of low-impact carbs a day.

Choose them from the list provided. You *must always* eat your carbs in the context of a meal, *with protein.* If you try eating three servings of low-impact carbs a day, and don't lose weight, try cutting back to one or two. If that still doesn't work for you— and remember, this is too much carb for my own personal body—you'll do better to try the Basic Low-Carbohydrate Diet, instead.

If you include one of the low-impact carbs with a meal and you're hungry and/or tired within ninety minutes or so, that particular carb isn't good for you. Try a different one and see how you react. And don't assume that you can substitute any old carbs for the ones on the list; you'll end up in trouble as sure as you were born. There is a *huge* difference between 100 percent whole grain rye bread from the health food store and commercial rye bread from the grocery store. The commercial kind is mostly "enriched" white flour and will spike your blood sugar just like white bread does. If you don't know for *sure* that a carb food has a low impact, *don't eat it!*

It is HIGHLY RECOMMENDED that you choose sweet carbs, *fruit included,* no more than once a day, and less is better. Despite the fact that fructose—fruit sugar—has a low glycemic index, it still has some not-so-great effects. It can cause high triglycerides, and some researchers feel that it stimulates fat formation more than any other kind of sugar. If you want more fruit than that, try cantaloupe, honeydew, strawberries, or raspberries, all of which are very low in total carbohydrates.

As you can see, this is the closest of any of these diets to being the traditional "balanced diet." Enough protein, probably more than you're used to eating, will give you energy and fill you up. The carbs that are allowed shouldn't trigger severe blood sugar swings, with their hunger and cravings and fatigue. Your insulin levels should stay moderate, though not as low as on the Basic Low-Carb Diet. And you'll be getting enough fat to make you feel satisfied, and to provide the essential fatty acids your body needs.

Interestingly, since I came up with this diet for Rob, Dr. Bob Arnot (medical dude for NBC News) has come out with his

Revolutionary Weight Control Program, which focuses on lean proteins and low-impact carbs! Not that far off from the Careful Carb Diet. My plan differs a bit from Dr. Arnot's—he feels that you should eat a fairly large amount of these low-impact carbs, especially beans. He also feels that you should avoid egg yolks and red meat and such, and that fat intake should be quite low. It's as if he's straddling two paradigms.

Personally, I'm convinced that for the vast majority of people, natural, unprocessed fats are harmless in moderate amounts; that for most of us, the yolk is the most nutritious part of the egg (not to mention the tastiest!); and, most importantly, that grains and beans are relative newcomers to the human diet, and that their safety in large quantity is highly suspect. But I see Dr. Arnot's diet as a big step in the right direction for the low-fat folks!

Game Rules for the Careful Carb Diet

1. You must consume your minimum protein requirement every day! Allowed proteins include meat, fish, poultry, eggs and eggs substitutes, cheese, and sugar-free protein powder. Eat a minimum of 14 grams of protein at breakfast. You must have protein at every meal, and you may divide up your protein so that you have snacks, too, if you like. Leaner proteins are better than fattier proteins—with the exception of fatty fishes such as salmon, mackerel, herring, and sardines, which are wonderful! Do not exceed your protein requirement by more than 20 grams a day.
2. Eat healthy fats in moderation, but do not use excessive quantities of added fat, or of very high-fat foods such as nuts and cheeses. A tablespoon or two of mayonnaise or olive oil is okay; half a cup is not!
3. Eat low-carbohydrate vegetables freely; the more the better. Low-carb veggies are:
    Alfalfa sprouts
    Artichokes
    Arugula
    Asparagus

Avocado

Beans
 (green, wax, and snap)

Beet greens

Bok choy

Broccoli

Brussels sprouts

Cabbage

Cauliflower

Celery

Chicory

Cucumber

Eggplant

Endive

Escarole

Kale

Lettuce (all kinds)

Mushrooms

Okra

Olives

Peppers

Pumpkin

Radishes

Sauerkraut

Spinach

Summer squash
 (zucchini, crookneck)

Turnip greens

Water Cress

4. Eat melons, berries, and borderline vegetables in moderation. Borderline vegetables are onions, garlic, rutabaga,
beets, spaghetti squash, turnips, tomatoes. As a guideline,
not more than half a large onion, or one large tomato, or a
couple of cloves of garlic at a meal.

5. Eat between one and three servings of the allowed
low-impact carbohydrate foods per day. Start with two
servings per day, and see how your hunger and your weight
react. If you're doing great, you may add one serving per
day. If you're not losing, and/or you're still hungry, drop
one serving a day. If you still have trouble, you may be so
severely carbohydrate intolerant that you'd do better on the
Basic Low-Carb Diet. Low-impact carbs must be eaten in
combination with proteins, not by themselves. DO NOT
eat any other concentrated carbohydrate foods!

Low-Impact Carbs
Grains and Other Starches

Whole grain barley (cook and use like rice) 1/2–3/4 cup

Steel cut oats (NOT rolled oats) 1/2–3/4 cup

Protein enriched pasta (Contadina makes a good one)
1/2–3/4 cup

DeBoles Jerusalem artichoke pasta 1/2–3/4 cup

Whole wheat pasta 1/2–3/4 cup

100% whole grain rye bread (no sugar, corn syrup, or
honey added) 1 small slice

Whole wheat pita (no sugar, corn syrup, or honey added—
many grocery stores have this) 1/2 round loaf

Yam or sweet potato 1 small

Peas 1/2–3/4 cup

Kidney beans 1/2–3/4 cup

Navy beans 1/2–3/4 cup

Butter beans 1/2–3/4 cup

Chickpeas 1/2–3/4 cup

Lentils 1/2–3/4 cup

Black beans 1/2–3/4 cup
(Oh, heck, all the dried beans except limas)

DO NOT eat canned baked beans or pork and beans—
they're loaded with sugar!

Hummus 1/2 cup

Winter squash (butternut, acorn, hubbard, spaghetti) 1/2 cup

All Bran, Fiber One, and other spaghetti-shaped bran
cereals 1/2 cup

Split pea, lentil, or bean soup 1 cup

Chili with beans (no sugar, corn syrup, or honey added)
1 cup

Hominy 1/2 cup

Brown rice 1/2 cup

Fruit

You already know which fruits are low-carb—berries, cantaloupe, honeydew.

Most other fruits may not be very low in carbohydrates, but they have a fairly low impact on blood sugar. Exceptions are kiwi, bananas, pineapple, raisins, grapes, and watermelon. Consider all other fruits to be okay low-impact carb choices. DO NOT EXCEED TWO FRUITS A DAY.

Other Low-Impact Carbs

> Milk 1 cup
> Tomato soup 1 cup
> Super-premium ice cream (Hagen Daaz, etc.)
>   NO CHUNKY VARIETIES 1/2 cup
> Peanut M&Ms 10–12 pieces
> Snickers 1 "fun size" bar (about 2″ long)
> All fruit-type jam or jelly 1 tablespoon

It is HIGHLY RECOMMENDED that you do NOT make all of your low-impact carb choices among the sweet carbs—that is, ice cream, M&Ms, Snickers, and fruit. This is NOT license to eat these things in an uncontrolled fashion!

6. Permitted beverages include tea; coffee; unsweetened sparkling waters, both plain and flavored; sugar-free soda; sugar-free fruit drinks.

7. You may have a glass of dry wine or a light beer with dinner. Read labels on light beers and look for one with 4 grams of carb or less per can or bottle—some "light" beers have as many as 11 grams per serving! Be aware that for some people, alcohol will prevent weight loss, and pay attention to your body. If you're not losing, you may need to trade one of your low-impact carbs for your drink, or abstain from alcohol altogether.

8. Avoid eating for entertainment! If you've had your breakfast at 7:30, and you're not hungry at noon, wait till you are hungry!

Typical Daily Menu for a Careful Carb Diet

BREAKFAST: Two eggs scrambled with peppers, mushrooms, and onions, stuffed in half a whole wheat pita
2˝ wedge cantaloupe
Coffee or tea

LUNCH: Chicken Caesar salad, no croutons
Iced tea, diet soda, or sugar-free fruit drink

DINNER: Cup of black bean soup
Pork chops, broiled with garlic and olive oil
Cole slaw with sugar-free dressing
Steamed broccoli with melted cheese
Light beer (less than 4 grams of carb per can)

SNACKS: Pork rinds, sunflower seeds, pumpkin seeds

Beyond the Glycemic Index

Remember the point I made several paragraphs back, that it was important to understand that the glycemic index tests involved eating whatever sized portion of the test food was needed to make up fifty grams of carbohydrate? This is the weakness of the whole concept of the glycemic index. Because of this particular point, some foods were made to appear taboo for the carbohydrate intolerant, when in reality, they could be tolerated in the sort of quantity that people generally eat them.

Carrots, it turns out, are a case in point. It is apparently true that eating enough carrots to consume 50 grams of carbohydrate will jack your blood sugar pretty high, but do you *know* how many carrots that is? More than fifty of those little baby carrots, that's how many. I don't know about you, but I don't like carrots that much! In other words, while half a cup of carrots contains more, and higher impact, carbohydrate than, say, half a cup of cucumber, they're not something we have to shun them altogether. For instance, when I make a pot of Sopa Azteca (wonderful Mexican soup!), I include, among other vegetables, one shredded carrot. Assuming that we call the whole potful six servings, that carrot adds a bit less than a gram of usable carbohydrate to each serving, and it surely improves the flavor and the vitamin content.

Enter the concept of the *glycemic load*.

"Glycemic load" is a new way of using those glycemic index tables to make them apply more realistically to food *as people actually eat it*. To calculate the glycemic load of a given food, you simply multiply the glycemic index of the food (using the white bread scale) by the number of grams of carbohydrate that are actually found in an average serving of that food. For instance: the glycemic index of soft drinks is about 97. There are about 42 grams of carbohydrate in a 12-ounce can of soda: .97 × 42 = 40.74, or something you *really* don't want to touch! Pumpernickel bread has a glycemic index of 71, and about 16 grams of carbohydrate per slice: .71 × 16 = 11.36; still pretty heavy duty. But while cooked carrots have a glycemic index of 56, a half-cup serving has only about 8.2 grams of carbohydrate: .56 × 8.2 = 4.6, or nowhere near as scary as either of our other examples.

(Why those decimal points? Because technically, that 100 at the top of the scale is really 1.00. So soda is really a 0.97, while pumpernickel is a 0.71. Hence the decimals.)

You can see the usefulness of this concept. The glycemic load gives us a real-world idea of what various foods are likely to do to our blood sugar and our bodies. It is interesting to note that the Harvard Nurses Study has looked at the glycemic load of the diets of the participants and has found that the risk of heart disease goes up with an increasing glycemic load.

Please keep in mind that none of this can tell you how much carbohydrate is appropriate for *your own body*. I know that I gain weight if I eat too much carbohydrate, *regardless of the source*. If you need to stay below, say, 60 grams a day, you need to stay below 60 grams a day, and the fact that those carbs have a more modest blood sugar impact won't keep you from gaining weight. Conversely, by sharply cutting your carb intake you are *dramatically* reducing your glycemic load, even if you were to get all of your very few grams of carb from sources with a high impact.

However, there is little question that you will do yourself a favor by choosing what few carbs you *do* eat from those with a modest glycemic index. And the day may not be too far off when officialdom scraps the dangerous food pyramid, and instead hands out daily glycemic load guidelines, and a big improvement it would be, too.

Indeed, the most encouraging thing to me about all this research on the importance of glycemic load is that the whole concept of limiting carbohydrate intake for health is becoming more and more accepted in the medical community.

For the most extensive list of glycemic indices I've been able to find, look online at http://www.mendosa.com/gilists.htm. This table gives the ratings both on the glucose scale and the white bread scale. To calculate glycemic load from these ratings, multiply the white bread scale number of the food in question by the number of grams of carbohydrate in a serving.

CHAPTER FIFTEEN

The Low-Carb Liquid Semi-Fast

A PERENNIALLY POPULAR approach to dieting is the replacement of meals with "diet shakes." From Metrecal and Slender in the 1960s to Ultra Slim-Fast today, many dieters like the idea of simply drinking most of their meals, partly for convenience's sake, partly for the easy portion control it offers, and partly because it lets them have something sweet a couple of meals a day!

Unfortunately, most of the diet shakes on the market today are as bad as they are overadvertised. The most highly advertised brand—*you* know which one—proudly crows that their shake provides "energy from carbohydrates," which is a sneaky way of saying that the stuff is simply *loaded* with sugar. You might just as well drink a fast food shake and take a vitamin pill! *(Don't you dare!)* If you're carb intolerant, ongoing use of these shakes can lead you into a nasty downward spiral, blood sugar crashing harder and harder, energy going lower and lower, getting more irritable by the day. And, of course, all your insulin-based health problems will worsen. Not good.

When I wrote the first edition of this book there was only one low-carb diet shake on the market, the Atkins shake. Now there are several, some tasting better than others. There are also Zone-inspired 30-30-40 shakes (and 30-30-40 bars). I still find them pretty expensive, and they have more sugar than I want.

If you don't mind the expense, low-carb diet shakes can be a useful tool in your weight-loss program. My sister, who has a slow metabolism and thus finds it quite hard to lose weight, has done very well drinking an Atkins shake for breakfast, another for lunch, and a third for a snack if she's really hungry. She then has a low-carb dinner of real food. This program, combined with walking a mile and a half most days, has helped her drop about thirty pounds in eight months. It also saves her all kinds of time making breakfast and a sack lunch!

But you don't *have* to use prepackaged shakes, if you'd prefer to make your own. Anyone who has a blender can make a diet shake! Dr. Michael Eades, of *Protein Power* fame, wrote a book in 1989 called *Thin So Fast,* in which he detailed a low-carbohydrate diet in which you drink homemade low-carb shakes three times a day and eat a low-carb meal of real food for dinner. His formula for the shakes calls for instant powdered milk, protein powder, a tiny amount of fructose, and some "lite salt" for the potassium. You combine these ingredients, then mix them with diet pop, sugar-free Kool-Aid, Crystal Light, whatever. I believe *Thin So Fast* is out of print, but any public library should be able to get it for you through Inter-Library Loan, if you'd like to read it. But as I've mentioned elsewhere, I'm a bit iffy about NutraSweet (aspartame). I don't drink many sugar-free beverages. I wanted a shake that didn't have artificial stuff in it.

Luckily, there's a completely natural carbohydrate and calorie-free sweetener available. It's called *stevia,* and it's an extract from the leaf of a Brazilian shrub. The Brazilian natives have used stevia leaves as a sweetener *forever,* and in Japan, everything that's sweetened with aspartame here, is sweetened with stevia instead. You can't buy food that's presweetened with stevia in the USA, but you can buy stevia itself and use it in things. The most common form is a white extracted powder, of which you use only very tiny quantities at a time. I pay $85.99 per pound for stevia in bulk at my health food store, which sounds expensive, but isn't. Since you use such small amounts, you don't need anything close to a pound! I bought a small jar for four or five bucks, and it's lasted for months. So stevia's not expensive to *use.*

There are a couple of other odd ingredients that are optional in this recipe: guar gum and xanthan gum. What the heck are these? Sounds icky! Actually, guar and xanthan are in lots of your favorite processed junk foods, so how horrible can they be? Guar and xanthan are both pure fiber, and they're very useful as thickeners. They add a nice texture to the shake without altering the flavor at all. Like stevia, guar and xanthan are used in tiny little quantities. The first time I experimented with guar, I did a one-for-one substitution for cornstarch—and it grabbed the spoon right out of my hand! I could have used the stuff to surface roads! I learned but *fast* to use guar and xanthan sparingly, and used that way, they're very helpful in replacing high-carb thickeners in our diet. You can get guar and xanthan at health food stores. They keep forever, and because you use so little at a time, they're not expensive. They do make the shakes nice and thick and creamy! Here's the recipe for your:

Basic Sugar-Free Protein Shake

- 1/3 cup instant dry skim milk
- 2 heaping tablespoons protein powder, or more if desired (This must be a protein powder with no carbohydrates. I recommend vanilla, which blends nicely with most other flavors, but unflavored protein powder will work fine. I like whey protein powder best.)
- 1 teaspoon cold pressed safflower oil (DON'T substitute inexpensive oil from the grocery; the label should read either "cold pressed" or "expeller pressed." Hain brand is good and has a very mild flavor. Store this in the refrigerator! You can leave out the oil if you add lecithin, flax seeds, or peanut butter.)
- 1/4 teaspoon white stevia extract powder, or more or less to taste. If you prefer, you can use artificial sweeteners.
- 3/4–1 cup cold water
- 3–5 ice cubes
- 1/4 teaspoon guar OR xanthan gum (Optional, but gives a thicker texture. Available at health food stores.)

Then you choose a flavoring. My favorite is a rounded table-spoon of unsweetened cocoa powder, plus a little instant coffee powder. My husband likes a heaping tablespoon of natural peanut butter, plus a little vanilla in his—but keep in mind that this adds both carbs (6 grams in 2 tablespoons of natural peanut butter) and substantial calories. If you're drinking two or three shakes a day, better go easy on the peanut butter. Berries are great in a shake—strawberries, raspberries, blueberries, what-ever. Use about half a cup. Again, this adds a few carbs, but also adds fiber and some potassium. Chocolate Raspberry or Chocolate Strawberry are both wonderful! You might like a cof-fee shake. Just add instant coffee powder, either regular or decaf, to taste—start with a scant teaspoonful, then taste as you go. If you like vanilla best, and didn't buy vanilla protein powder, add at least a good teaspoon of real vanilla extract. You can make a vanilla shake taste richer by adding a smidge of salt, too, and a little cinnamon or nutmeg might be nice!

Of course, your grocery store offers scads of flavorings and extracts for you to play around with. How about adding a drop of mint extract to a chocolate shake to get chocolate mint? Or how about rum extract? Orange? Almond? No need to get bored—but to be honest, I usually make good old chocolate!

You can, if you like, add extra nutritional ingredients to your shake; I often do. For instance, I usually add *lecithin*. This is a substance found in egg yolks and soybeans that is used as an *emulsifier*—that is, to make oil and water combine. It's the lecithin in egg yolk that makes mayonnaise and hollandaise sauce thicken and hold together. Lecithin is also what makes nonstick cooking spray work. It's quite nutritious, good for your nerves, brain, and skin, and for lowering cholesterol. Lecithin also has a reputation for helping even out fat distribu-tion on your body, and improving fat burning. Whether this last is true, I have no concrete evidence, but I know it's good for me, and it improves the texture of the shake—makes it very creamy—without changing the flavor, so I usually add a big tablespoon of the stuff. By the way, you'll find lecithin at your health food store, in liquid, capsules, or granules. The granules are what you want for shakes—the liquid is as thick as 40-weight on a January day. Store 'em in the fridge.

Another thing I sometimes add is *bee pollen*. This is, of course, the male reproductive part of flowers, and is *loaded* with vitamins, minerals, protein, enzymes, phytonutrients, and such. It has a little carb in it, but so much nutrition that it seems worth it to me. Don't buy dried bee pollen or tablets. Look for a store that sells fresh bee pollen granules and stores them in the cooler. Unlike lecithin and guar, bee pollen does have a flavor, but the flavor is just sort of mildly sweet and flowery. I use maybe a heaping teaspoon per shake. And, of course, if you have a severe pollen allergy, you'd want to be very, very careful if you tried pollen, right? (Some people claim that eating bee pollen, starting with just a grain or two, will build up an immunity and get rid of the allergy. I have *no idea* if this is true or not. I'd be *very* careful. Or just leave it out altogether.)

You can also add flax seeds to a shake! These will add thickness—flax seeds are *loaded* with fiber—and also will add very healthy oil. Flax seeds, as I mentioned before, are an excellent source of the same healthy fats you get in fish. They can help with inflammation and pain, lower cholesterol and blood pressure, and there's some evidence that they help with fat burning. Of course, the fiber will help with any irregularity you might have. Flax seeds will grind up in the shake if you run the blender long enough; I haven't noticed that they hurt the flavor much. Up to you! I'd use about a tablespoon.

Then there are two things I sometimes add a *tiny* amount of. I add them because they're very, very nutritious, but I add tiny amounts because they taste *god-awful*. I wouldn't mind at all if you left them out, but I often add just a scant teaspoon of nutritional yeast (loaded with B vitamins and minerals), and maybe an eighth of a teaspoon of spirulina, a very nutritious algae. Both of these are available at health food stores, but if you have really sensitive taste buds, these may not be for you.

Anyway, put the water in the blender *first*. This will help prevent the dry ingredients from caking at the bottom. Then add all your dry ingredients, your flavorings, extra nutritional stuff, etc.

Turn on the blender, and drop in the ice cubes, *one at a time*. I like to let my shake whip at high speed for a few minutes; it makes it pretty thick. Speaking of which, people often ask if they can just use a cup of fluid skim milk instead, and the answer is yes, but the powdered skim whips up better for some strange reason. I think it's a lot better. It's cheaper, too, and easier to store.

Depending on what you use to flavor the shake, it will have somewhere in the neighborhood of 15 to 20 grams of carbohydrate, most of it from the milk. Fortunately, lactose has a fairly modest impact on blood sugar levels and shouldn't cause a major crash. So long as you're not *terribly* carb sensitive, and keep your intake of carbs from other sources very low, this shouldn't be a problem. Depending on your protein powder, your shake should have 25 to 30 grams of protein, enough to keep you going for *hours*. And unless you use peanut butter or another high-fat flavoring, it will be quite low in calories, too. (Still, peanut oil is a healthy fat. If you like peanut butter shakes, use natural peanut butter, not Skippy or Jif, which have hydrogenated oil and sugar in them! If using peanut butter in your shake fills you up for longer, and you need one less shake a day, then you can have a *few* more carbs with your dinner!)

You can use one of these shakes as an occasional meal replacement, if you like. I drink them for lunch fairly often. If you're on the Basic Low-Carb Diet, you'll have to subtract the carbohydrate grams from some other meal, of course. The shakes don't really fit into the Carb Controlling program, since they aren't low carb enough for a low-carb meal, and why would you have one at your Reward Meal?

A good use of shakes is for breakfast, as my sister Kim is fond of doing. If you're one of those folks who just can't handle cooked food in the morning, a shake is perfect for you! And if you put all the stuff, except the ice cubes of course, in the blender jar the night before, and store it overnight in the refrigerator, you can then throw in the ice, turn on the blender, go brush your hair or throw on your clothes, and breakfast will be ready to go. You can even drink it in the car. Hey, make a coffee shake and you won't even have to slow down to drink your coffee!

If you're one of the minority who have the 50/50 cholesterol reaction to low carbing that I mentioned earlier—your triglycerides go down and your HDL goes up, which is good, but your LDL goes up, too, which is bad—shakes can be a very good idea for you, because they're an easy way to get flax seed, for its heart-healthy fats and fiber, and a heaping tablespoon of lecithin, for its cholesterol-dissolving properties.

But the real value of the shakes, either purchased or homemade, is this: If you like a simple, shake-based diet because it's a no-brainer, you can drink two or three of these shakes during the day, and you'll feel full, have high energy, and be getting both reasonably low carbs *and* low calories—again, a hybrid diet— and, depending on what extras you add, a *ton* of nutrition as well. (You can take a homemade shake to work in a thermos for lunch, of course. Shake it up well before you open the thermos. Or, you can take a store-bought shake in a can or bottle.) Then—and this is *essential*—for dinner you *must* have a low-carb dinner of *both* meat, fish, poultry, or eggs *and* plenty of low-carb vegetables. This is to supply the nutrients that are missing from the shake. Since you're getting a fair amount of low-impact carbs in the shake, keep your dinner very low carb, okay?

Since you're not eating as much "real food" on this program, you should be very careful to take your vitamins every day, and also to take a potassium supplement, unless you take potassium-sparing blood pressure medication. If you're on this sort of medication, CONSULT YOUR DOCTOR AND PHARMACIST before taking a supplement.

CHAPTER SIXTEEN

Low Carb for Vegetarians

VEGETARIANS WHO HAVE read this far are thinking, "How the heck can I do this? All that meat! I guess low carb just isn't for me." Yet you may have recognized yourself in the list of the symptoms of carbohydrate intolerance. So, is it possible to be a low-carb vegetarian?

Yes, it is, and I can give you some pointers on how to do it.

However, I would first like to suggest that, if you've become a vegetarian for health reasons, you reconsider that decision. You don't have to eat piles of red meat if you don't want to. There's still some controversy over whether or not unlimited quantities of red meat are great for you. But you might consider adding at least fish, and possibly poultry, back to your diet. I've known *many* vegetarians who, having done this, found that they feel a *lot* better.

If, on the other hand, your decision to be a vegetarian is a moral one, I cannot and will not argue with that. You must, of course, follow the dictates of your own conscience.

That being said, let's take a look at low-carb nutrition for vegetarians.

It's protein that's the problem, of course. There's a piece of "wisdom" traveling around in vegetarian—and especially in vegan—circles that says that you really don't need much protein, that your body really requires only 30 to 45 grams of protein a day, and that if you're getting enough calories, you're getting enough protein.

This all depends, of course, on what your definition of "enough" is. You'll probably get enough protein to stave off killing malnutrition; you probably won't end up with kwashior-kor (that awful bloated-belly syndrome that you see in starving children). This says nothing about the amount of protein needed for optimal health, and even less about the amount of protein needed by a person who is eating very few carbohydrates, and who therefore needs to consume an extra margin of protein to fuel gluconeogenesis to supply what little carbohydrate his or her body really needs. (You remember, gluconeogenesis is the process by which your body makes carbohydrates from proteins and, a little bit, from fats. This, of course, applies only to vegetarians who decide that they feel best on a very low-carb, ketogenic diet. If you choose a less carb-restricted diet, you won't need protein for gluconeogenesis.) Low-carb vegetarians should be aiming for the same protein intake as nonvegetarian low carbers—2 grams per each pound of healthy body weight per day.

So, that being said, let's have a little....

Protein 101

Proteins are made up of amino acids, in very much the same way words are made up of letters. You eat protein, your body breaks it down into those individual "letters," and then, in a huge, physiological game of Scrabble, it reassembles those "letters" into all the different "words" and "sentences," or types of protein, your body needs. Every protein in your body, from your skin and hair and nails to your liver and spleen and antibodies, is "spelled" from different combinations of those amino acids. Many of those amino acids your body can actually make from *other* amino acids—sort of like if you had a Scrabble letter *A*, scratched out the crossbar, turned it upside down, and had a *V*. But there are nine amino acids that your body can't make—it *must* get them from your food. These are called "essential amino acids." It's not that your body needs them more than the others, but rather that it is essential for your body to get them *from your food*.

To continue with our spelling metaphor, think of these essential amino acids as being the vowels—you simply can't make words without them, even if you have all the other letters. In just this way, if you have all the amino acids, even *most* of the essential ones, but you're missing just one or two of these essential amino acids, your body will not be able to "spell" the protein words and sentences needed to repair itself—and will begin breaking down your muscles to get the missing amino acids! So it is *vital* that you consume all of these amino acids *every day*.

Animal proteins—meat, eggs, and dairy products—contain all of the essential amino acids in the proper balance necessary for your body to be able to "spell" all the different proteins it needs. To use the Scrabble example yet again, your body needs more of some amino acids, and less of others, just like you need more *E*s and fewer *Q*s to play Scrabble. Plant foods are nearly always short on one amino acid or another. This is the reason why vegetarians are encouraged, for instance, to combine grains with beans: because each has essential amino acids that the other lacks. The combination of the two gives you all of the essential amino acids in the right quantities, much like an animal protein would. This is also why soy products have been considered a superior plant source of protein—the balance of the various amino acids is closer to that of animal foods than any other vegetable protein source. However, as I'll explain in a minute, there are compelling reasons not to eat unlimited quantities of soy products.

Most vegetarians are accustomed to getting much of their protein from combinations of beans and grains, and while it is quite true that these combine to make protein of a quality as good as that of animal foods, they carry *vast* amounts of carbohydrate along with them. If you're carbohydrate intolerant, you simply cannot afford to eat piles of starch to get your protein.

Depending on how carbohydrate intolerant you are, however, you may be able to keep *some* grains and beans in your diet. For instance, you could try the Carb Controlling approach, and eat your grains and beans at dinner, along with a big salad and a low-carb vegetable—but if you do this, I'd strongly suggest that you not eat a dessert as well; you'll be getting all the carbohydrate that even a Reward Meal can bear from the main course. Or you could try the Careful Carb Diet, which would allow you one to three small servings of low-impact carbs a day. You would then choose those low-impact carbs from the bean and grain products listed in that chapter (for example, a cup of black bean soup with lunch, and half a whole wheat pita with dinner). But in neither of these cases would you be getting any-where *near* enough protein from those grains and beans. And some of you will find that you're *so* carbohydrate intolerant that even at this reduced level of consumption, those grains and beans are keeping you fat, hungry, and tired. Either way, you're going to need another, lower-carb source of quality protein.

There was a time when I recommended that vegetarians simply turn to soy foods for their protein. I can no longer, in good conscience, make that recommendation. Soy is not the same critter today as the *glycine soya* that Asian cultures domesticated between 500 and 1,000 years ago. (This, by the way, makes soy one of the newest additions to the human diet, even if it hadn't been *seriously* hybridized, which it has.) It's been bred to have higher levels of hormones, apparently because those estrogens help fatten cattle (what do they do to us?), and the bean has been changed so much it has a new name: *glycine max*. All those extra hormones, which are being sold to us as a tremendous health boon, may not be so great after all. As I mentioned a minute ago, there are too many unhappy consequences of unlimited soy consumption coming to light. What unhappy consequences?

- A British study published in 2000 showed a fivefold greater risk for a specific genital birth defect of boy babies in vege-tarian mothers. The reason has not been established, but scientists suspect the problem is the high level of estrogens from soy in vegetarian diets. The particular defect is called "hypospadias"—the urethra is too short, and exits the penis along the base of the penis, rather than at the tip.
- A 1999 study in Hawaii turned up the worrisome fact that middle-aged men who ate two or more servings of tofu per week had an increased risk of brain deterioration in old age.

The greater the tofu consumption, the greater the cognitive impairment. Again, this is not firmly established—just because two things happen together doesn't mean that the one causes the other—but it is pretty darned scary. The speculation is that the estrogens in the tofu bind to receptors in the brain meant for the body's own estrogen, causing the problems. If this is, indeed, the case, all soy foods that contain a lot of isoflavones (soy estrogens) would be a risk.

- Despite the reputation soy has for preventing breast cancer, there's some evidence that in women who already have breast cancer, soy can cause faster tumor growth. Keep in mind that a low-carb diet appears to be a pretty good defense against breast cancer in and of itself.
- Soy has been known for a long time to cause thyroid dysfunction, including goiter and—in some cases—autoimmune thyroid disease. The last thing you need if you're trying to lose weight, become more energetic, and improve your health is a malfunctioning thyroid gland.
- Soy contains substances called phytates, which interfere with mineral absorption. Phytates are present in other grains and beans as well, but in many foods, processing and cooking break them down. This is not so with the phytates in soy foods. As a result, a diet high in soy can cause mineral deficiencies.
- The FDA refused to grant soy protein isolate GRAS (Generally Recognized As Safe) status, partly because of concerns about thyroid problems, and partly because it felt that Archer Daniels Midland (the big agribusiness company that is the largest soybean producer) had not been forthcoming with evidence that the protein isolate was safe.

So you can see why I can't recommend you eat a lot of soy. However, it's good to know that *fermented* soy foods—tempeh, miso, and natto—appear to be safer, because much of the phytoestrogen content is destroyed during fermentation. It is also interesting to note that these fermented soy foods have accounted, historically, for much of the soy consumption in countries where soy is traditionally eaten. However, unlike the more concentrated tofu, soy protein powder, soy cheese, and soy meat analogues, these fermented soy foods have more carbohydrate than protein. Keep this in mind if you use them. (By the way, soy sauce falls into this category of fermented soy foods, too, but is not a source of protein.)

So if you're not eating tofu and soy cheese, where will you get your protein?

If you're a lacto-ovo vegetarian, you can eat cheese, eggs, and yogurt. These three foods are infinitely versatile and can provide you with plenty of high-quality protein, with very little carbohydrate. An omelet for breakfast, vegetables with a yogurt-based dip or a salad with grated cheese and chopped hard-boiled eggs for lunch, and—depending on the degree of your carbohydrate intolerance—either a Reward Meal of grains and beans or a tempeh stir-fry without rice for dinner should keep you full and energetic all day long. In addition, there are many wonderful recipes combining cheese or eggs or both with vegetables that make elegant main dishes for a low-carbohydrate lacto-ovo vegetarian.

Another *terrific* option for vegetarian low carbers is to keep low-carb baked goods made from whey protein powder on hand. Whey protein is of excellent quality, plus in most of these recipes it will be combined with eggs, as well, making these baked goods as good a source of protein as meat, poultry, or fish. My cookbook, *500 Low-Carb Recipes,* has quite a few recipes that are made this way. I also heartily recommend that you buy the two low-carb baking books by my friend Diana Lee, *Baking Low Carb* and *Bread and Breakfast: Baking Low Carb II.* Actually, I recommend these books for all low carbers, but for vegetarians they're even more important. With these books in hand (and a modest stock of specialty ingredients), you can be getting your protein from muffins, zucchini bread, granola, even French toast made from low-carb bread. These foods do include some carbohydrate, which, of course, you will have to count—but the level of variety they bring to a low-carb vegetarian diet is wonderful.

The rest of your diet will, of course, consist of the same low-carb vegetables, low-sugar fruits, nuts, seeds, and healthy fats that all low-carbers eat.

But what about the low-carb vegan? Is low-carb veganism even possible? Without access to the sort of money I'd need for major research, the best I can do is make an educated guess. But, hey, since when did that ever stop me?

I suspect that low-carb veganism is possible, but *not* desirable. A vegan diet is *always* a nutritional compromise. There is no question that humankind evolved eating animal foods, and we absolutely *require* one vitamin that is *only* found in animal foods, B12. (There has been speculation that some fermented soy foods contain B12; this appears to be untrue.) And there are other nutrients that, although found in plant foods, are in their most accessible forms in animal foods. This is true of both calcium and iron, for instance. (I'm not speaking of dairy calcium, here, but rather of calcium from bones. This appears to be the most highly absorbable calcium there is.)

So, if you are a vegan for nutritional reasons, I urge you to widen your diet to include at least eggs and dairy products. However, once again, if you are a vegan for moral or spiritual reasons, I cannot and will not argue with you. To be a moral vegan with severe carbohydrate intolerance must be a very uncomfortable place to be; I'll see if I can make it a little easier.

First of all, forget the nonsense you've read about how you can get lots of protein from vegetables. This is simply false. The highest-protein vegetables—this would include things like broccoli, asparagus, artichokes, and avocados—have about 2 to 4 grams of protein per serving. You'd have to do virtually nothing all day but sit around shoveling in vegetables to get anything *approaching* enough protein from these vegetables—and even with these low-carb vegetables, you'd be getting too much carbohydrate this way.

Even eating that many vegetables, there would be no guarantee that the protein you got would be of adequate quality. How, then, is a low carber who eats no animal foods at all to get enough high-quality protein? It is a puzzle, no?

What *can* vegan low carbers eat?

Nuts and seeds. And more nuts and seeds. And even more nuts and seeds! And, I might add, more seeds than nuts. Sunflower seeds and pumpkin seeds have more protein in them, ounce for ounce, than any of the tree nuts—almonds, pecans, walnuts, hazelnuts, Brazil nuts, etc. Sesame seeds are also a good one to use, although they're awfully small to eat in a mix!

The different nuts and seeds have differing quantities of those essential amino acids, so you will want to eat a variety—and eat a variety *daily*. In other words, don't eat sunflower seeds today, almonds tomorrow, hazelnuts the next day, and pumpkin seeds later in the week. Eat all of these, each day. You don't have to eat them at exactly the same time for your body to be able to use the amino acids, but you do have to eat them within a few hours of each other. It's best to buy or make nut-and-seed mix, using plenty of pumpkin and sunflower seeds plus a variety of the tree nuts.

The vegan low carber will likely also want to make at least some use of the fermented soy products mentioned—a cup of miso soup, a salad with a scattering of toasted sesame seeds or sunflower seeds, and a few handfuls of nut-and-seed mix would be a reasonable meal for a vegan low carber.

Using various nut butters is also a good idea for the vegetarian and vegan low carber. It's important that you not limit yourself to the familiar peanut butter; its amino acid profile is inadequate by itself. Tahini—roasted sesame paste—is an important food for you, and so are sunflower butter and almond butter. A *brilliant* thing to do is to combine several of these into a mixed nut-and-seed butter; this will have a *far* better nutritional profile than any of these butters alone. Of course, without bread, you'll have to figure out ways to eat this other than in sandwiches! You can, of course, spread nut butters on fiber crackers. You could also make nut butter-based sauces—similar to the Asian peanut sauce—to go over vegetables. And you can stuff celery stalks! You'll need to become a creative cook, no doubt about it. (Or you could just eat your nut butter with a spoon, right out of the jar. This is what my husband does!)

You could, of course, use vegetarian protein powder, but many of these are made from soy protein isolate, which, as we've already mentioned, has not been proclaimed safe by the FDA. I've tried a soy-free vegetarian protein powder made from mixed sources, including peas, and it was just plain nasty. I can't recommend it. The best-tasting soy-free vegetarian protein powder I've found—it is simply very bland, much like flour —is Rice Protein Powder by NutriBiotic, of Lakeland, California. If your health food store doesn't have it, see if they can special order it for you, or go online to www.nutribiotic.com for more information on where to get it.

A couple of things to keep in mind about the Rice Protein Powder: First of all, it does contain some carbs, which you'll need to count. Second, NutriBiotic is very clear that their Rice Protein has the same amino acid profile as the protein you would derive by eating rice—it just has most of the carbohydrates removed. This means that it is an *unbalanced protein,* low in some of the essential amino acids, just as rice is, and will need to be consumed *with other vegetable proteins* to be fully utilized by the body. One good use for it might be to make vegan nut-and-seed balls—combine natural peanut butter, tahini, almond butter, and sunflower butter, then blend in Splenda or stevia to sweeten (you could add a little vanilla, if you like) and enough Rice Protein Powder to make a stiff, almost crumbly paste. Roll into balls, and eat for snacks. This should yield protein of an excellent quality.

And I'm afraid that's about it for low-carb sources of complete vegan protein: Fermented soy products, nuts and seeds, vegetarian soy-free protein powder. I don't know of any reason why you couldn't be fairly healthy on these things, but you might get very bored, very fast. The suggestion that you try the Carb Controlling or Careful Carb diets goes double for the vegan, for this very simple reason of staving off boredom.

I would also suggest that low-carb vegetarians take some real pains to come up with truly interesting vegetable dishes, both hot and cold. This will be one of the great sources of variety and interest in these narrower versions of a low-carb diet.

My last thought on the subject is this: Believing that killing animals for food is wrong does not change what your body needs. Morality cannot shift the weight of millions of years of dietary evolution. You must follow the dictates of your conscience, but do so with your eyes open, and with careful thought to overcoming the nutritional problems that can result for those of us whose bodies cannot cope with a lot of carbohydrate.

Be well!

CHAPTER SEVENTEEN

Wrapping It Up

S O THERE ARE the diets. And now that you've read through them all, you should have a pretty good grip of the basics of low-carb dieting: Get enough protein, eat only healthy fats, treat carbohydrates with extreme caution. You'll want to choose one of these approaches and try it for a few weeks or months, and see how it fits you—your personality, your body, your lifestyle. If one doesn't fit you quite right, try another! That's why I haven't given you a one-size-fits-all diet plan. I want you to find the path that's right for you; the Way of Eating that will see you through a healthy lifetime.

Further, there's no reason you can't mix and match to find what's best for you, so long as you're *very* careful about keeping your carb load low. For instance, you could try doing a Carb Controlling approach where you eat only low-impact carbs at your Reward Meal, for a faster weight loss, better control of your hunger, and faster improvement of your blood work. If you entertain a lot on the weekends, and want to be able to eat all the foods you cook for others, you could do the Basic Low-Carb Diet or the Liquid Semi-Fast during the week, and then switch to a Carb Controlling diet on the weekends—or you could serve only low-impact carbs at your dinner parties! You could do a Cyclic Ketogenic Diet where you use only low-impact carbs during your carb-up. You could do a Cyclic Ketogenic Diet where you do a carb-up only when you stop going into ketosis easily, then carb up for three or four days before heading back into ketosis for another month or two. Or, as I sometimes do, you could do a Basic Low-Carb Diet most of the year, and switch over to a Paleolithic Diet when the fruit is ripe in the summer, to sneak in a few more cherries and nectarines.

Something you should absolutely *not* do is combine the Careful Carb Diet with the Carb Controlling Diet —eating low-impact carbs all day, and then having a Reward Meal with lots more carbs—even high-impact carbs—once a day. You'll be sorry if you do! If you're eating the Carb Controlling Diet, you don't ever get to do the twelve- to twenty-four-hour carb-up from the Cyclic Ketogenic Diet, either! You may be able to fool yourself, but you can't fool your body.

That being said, the vast majority of Americans would *dramatically* improve their health, sense of well-being, appearance, and waistlines if they simply quit eating anything with refined, processed, valueless carbohydrates—sugar and corn syrup, white flour products, cold cereals, all that garbage—ate their vegetables and healthy fats, and made sure they got enough protein at every meal.

The point is, I want you to understand the *principles* so you have tools to work with. With all these different approaches, I think you have those tools.

In review, here's a quick rundown of the basics of taming your runaway insulin and losing weight permanently:

1. Be afraid—be VERY afraid!—of added sugar in all forms: sugar, corn syrup, malt syrup, fruit juice concentrate, honey, molasses, brown sugar, maple syrup, Sucanat, turbinado, fructose, dextrose, maltose, or anything else ending in -ose. THERE IS NO SUCH THING AS "GOOD SUGAR." (Many products labeled "No sugar added" have honey, fruit juice, or malt syrup. These are sugar!) Be wary even of the natural sugars in fruits. Remember: If it tastes even a little bit sweet, and it isn't artificially sweetened, it's got some kind of sugar! (Exception: There are now many sugar-free products out there—candy, ice cream, you name

it—that use polyols, also known as sugar alcohols. You'll know these sweeteners by the "ol" in their name—maltitol, sorbitol, lactitol, xylitol, etc. We'll talk about these in a later chapter—they're sort of controversial.)

2. Avoid grains, including bread, crackers, rice, pasta, cereal, pizza crust, biscuits, muffins, etc.
    Avoid dried beans and other starchy legumes, and starchy or sugary vegetables such as potatoes, corn, peas, and carrots. IF YOU WISH TO BREAK THIS RULE, IT IS BEST TO EAT THE LEAST-PROCESSED, HIGHEST-FIBER, HIGHEST-NUTRIENT CARBOHYDRATES THAT YOU CAN. Coarsely ground whole grain rye bread, steel cut oats, and homemade black bean soup will cause you far less harm than white flour bagels, sugary cold cereal, and (corn-syrup laced) canned pork and beans. We won't even talk about rubbish like marshmallow squares and fake canned biscuits.

3. The more strictly you are willing to cut out carbohydrates, the less you will have to concern yourself with portion control or calories. If you wish to keep some of the less damaging carbs in your diet, you may well have to control portions and/or limit calories as well. There are some hard choices to be made here, make them with your eyes wide open!

4. Eat plenty of unprocessed, carb-free protein foods. Eat protein at every meal. If you choose to eat a carbohydrate food, eat protein with it. Protein is the cornerstone of your diet, all other foods are secondary. Eating your protein will increase your metabolism and keep you feeling full and energetic longer than any other kind of food.

5. Eat only fresh, unprocessed, natural fats. Don't use polyunsaturated oils for cooking—safflower, soy, corn, sunflower, etc.; they break down rapidly and become unhealthy when heated. Olive, canola, coconut, and peanut oils are all right for cooking, as are butter and fresh meat fats (chicken fat, pork fat—don't use purchased lard, it's heavily processed and hydrogenated). Do not eat

margarine, vegetable shortening, or other "hydrogenated" fats. DO NOT TRY TO EAT A LOW-CARB DIET THAT IS ALSO LOW IN FAT.

6. Get plenty of high-fiber, low-carb foods, especially low-carb vegetables. Nuts and seeds are excellent foods, high in fiber, protein, minerals, and valuable fats, but they are also very high in calories, so eat them with at least a bit of restraint if you're having trouble losing weight. With almost all of these plant foods, raw or only lightly cooked is best.

7. Eat a high-protein breakfast every day. If you're not hungry when you get up, take some protein food to work with you, to eat in the car or at your first break. And stop eating so heavily at night! If you eat less at night, you'll wake up with an appetite. Why lay in a bunch of food just before going to sleep?

8. Drink plenty of water!

9. Learn to listen to your hunger, which on a low-carb diet you should be able to trust. I didn't say this elsewhere, but it's important to point out: Americans have been trained to munch mindlessly for hours on carb-y junk food that never fills them up—what I call the "hand-to-mouth routine." There's very little in the way of low-carb food that you can do this with, for the very simple reason that low-carb foods are filling. The big exception, of course, is very low carb vegetables, which you may munch on to your heart's content. Other "entertainment" foods are sunflower seeds or pumpkin seeds in the shell. Because you have to crack each shell and each kernel is so small, it's hard to eat too many. (I sneak sunflower seeds into the movies with me!) Pork rinds are no carb—unless you get them barbeque style or with other flavors, READ THE LABEL—and mostly air, so you can munch on these, too. (Personally, I reach my pork rind limit after about four. But some people adore the things.) If you try to eat most low-carb foods—meat, poultry, fish, cheese, nuts, eggs—endlessly, you'll make yourself sick to your stomach! (A sugar-junkie was at my house

one day, uninvited, and wanted me to feed her lunch when I was busy. I threw her a bag of nut-and-seed mix. That afternoon, she complained of being nauseated. When I picked up the bag of nut-and-seed mix later on and discovered she'd eaten well over a pound of the stuff, I understood why she felt sick!) Again, learn to listen to your hunger.

10. Read the labels on everything you put into your body. Most people do far more research before buying a car or a VCR than they do on what they put into their own bodies. "You are what you eat" is literally true. All your body has to make itself from is what you put in your mouth. If you give your body junk, you'll be made out of junk, and you'll feel and look like it.

11. Make the best choice possible given any particular circumstance. What do I mean? If you're at work and the vending machine has cookies, crackers, chips, candy, and peanuts, the peanuts are the best choice, even though they're relatively high carb for a nut (because, of course, they're really a legume!). When you're genuinely hungry, and faced with foods that are not ideal for the diet, choose the food that will screw you up the least. Don't be afraid to pick off breading, eat only the cheese and toppings off the pizza, ask for an extra salad in place of the potato, etc.

12. Buy a food counter book, one that lists not only carbohydrates and calories, but also fiber, so you can subtract the grams of fiber from the grams of carbohydrate. If you're not absolutely certain that a food is low in carbs, LOOK IT UP! You can also use the USDA Nutrient Database, at http://www.nal.usda.gov/fnic/cgi-bin/nut_search.pl. That's a mighty cumbersome URL, so why don't you put it on your "favorites" or "bookmarks" list? It's a wonderful resource.

13. Take a high-quality, broad-spectrum multiple vitamin and mineral supplement every day. This should be a supplement that requires that you take more than one tablet a day—six is not excessive, depending on how big or small a tablet you can swallow.

Don't Become Dependant on the Scale!

One other tip—don't become too dependant on your scale. Yes, we've been talking all along about "weight loss," but now might be an appropriate time to mention that weighing yourself is actually a pretty lame way to determine how fat you are. Why? Because a scale weighs all of you, fat and muscle, bones and blood, and skin and hair. How do you know what part of you is getting heavier or lighter?

To put it another way, if you wanted to buy the leanest steak in the grocery store, you wouldn't just pick the lightest one, would you? Of course not.

Or, think of it this way: Arnold Schwartzenegger is heavier than average for his height. Do you think he's fat? For that matter, I'm still fairly heavy for a woman of my height and percent body fat, largely because I'm quite muscular, and muscle weighs much more than fat. (For this very reason, you may gain a pound or two if you start working out. Don't panic; you're exchanging fat for muscle, a good bargain no matter how you look at it!)

So use your scale, but don't consider it the ultimate judge of how fat or slim you are, or whether you're losing fat. Here's a better way: Most of us have on hand some piece of clothing that doesn't fit us anymore—something we've kept, hoping to fit back into it someday. Jeans are probably the best. Try on that too-small pair of jeans, or dress, or whatever. Then try it on again each week as you diet. See how much closer you are to being able to fasten it. At first, the zipper may be five inches apart in front. Then four inches. Then three. One day, you can fasten the button! Pretty exciting.

Or, you can use a belt, and see where it fastens each week. If you use an old one, you can mark it with a magic marker to show your progress. Or you can be truly revolutionary and use a tape measure!

It's not uncommon, by the way, for inch loss to occur even when weight loss does not. In fact, I've talked with a few low carbers who find that when they're losing pounds, their size stays pretty much the same. Then their weight will plateau for a week or so, but they'll be losing inches all the while. Odd, but true. It's also common to not lose any weight—or even go up a pound or two—for a week or so when your menstrual period is due, only to then have a goodish drop in weight when it starts. This is sometimes known as the "whoosh," or even "a visit from the Whoosh Fairy"!

In any case, pay attention to what *size* you are, in addition to what you *weigh*. It's a far more accurate way to gauge your progress.

CHAPTER EIGHTEEN

The Indulgence

NOW, LET'S TALK about a very important subject:

CHEATING!

I'm not naive. I know you're going to cheat! It's a-gonna happen. You know it, I know it. So let's talk about it here and now! After all, a good offense is the best defense.

In fact, I *plan* to cheat—and that's what I want you to do. I don't even call it cheating. I call it an "Indulgence."

I like this term far better, because the word "cheating" implies that you're going to get away with something. I remember my father coming into the kitchen an hour after dinner and eating ice cream out of the container. He'd get this look on his face that screamed, "Aren't I a cute, mischievous little boy? Look what I'm getting away with!" But he didn't get away with a thing. He was fat. And he was hospitalized with heart disease at the age of fifty-five. *There is no cheating; you can't fool your body. You don't get away with a thing.*

So, don't even try to cheat. Plan to Indulge, instead. Then *you* have the power!

How often do I have an Indulgence? Not as often as you might think! As I revise this chapter, I haven't had a sugar-sweetened dessert for over a year and a half. Pretty good, huh? But I've reached this place after *eight years* of low carbing.

I'm not deliberately being good; I've just reached a blessed state of not caring about carbohydrate foods! I lost interest quite a while ago—especially since I know so many wonderful low-carb treats! Example: Three years after I started low carbing, I went to a huge wedding over Memorial Day weekend, and had every intention of eating a dessert at the reception. They had a fabulous sweets table, so there were all kinds of choices—but I was too busy dancing to slow myself down with sugar. I just never got around to it. If you had asked me as a kid if I would ever be having too good a time to get around to eating sugar, I would have thought you were nuts!

You're not at that point yet. So think ahead. What are the times when it will really, I mean *really*, be important to you to eat carbs? The holidays spring to mind. I eat whatever I want on Thanksgiving Day and Christmas Day. And I expect you to do the same! You might want to add your birthday to the list of Indulgence days. How about your anniversary? Give yourself between five and eight occasions during the year—and they don't have to be fixed occasions like holidays. If you're going to a party and you know the host is a marvelous cook, you might choose to make that one of your Indulgences. Or maybe you're going on vacation and know that you'll be visiting a five-star restaurant. Indulgence time!

But! Remember there is *danger* here! I spoke to a small club of low-carb dieters in my town, and one woman said she *had* to eat cake that night because it was her daughter's birthday. It is all very well to decide that *your* birthday is an Indulgence day. It is quite another thing to decide that *everyone's* birthday is an Indulgence day! If you have an Indulgence on your birthday, your husband's birthday, your mother's birthday, your father's birthday, your sister's birthday, your brother's birthday, each of your kids' birthdays, your officemates' birthdays, you're not having an Indulgence, you're fooling yourself. And you'll stay fat, tired, and sick.

Likewise, there is a HUGE difference between deciding that on Thanksgiving Day and Christmas Day you may have an Indulgence, and deciding that "It's the Holiday season," so you can make like a Hoover at all the holiday parties and cookie exchanges for the whole month from Thanksgiving till Christmas. If you do that, you'll be shopping the post-Christmas sales for new clothes in a larger size!

Beware the lesser holidays! If you have an Indulgence every time Hallmark comes out with new cards, you'll never get there! Groundhog Day, St. Patrick's Day, Columbus Day—these don't count! And it's one thing to have chocolate on Valentine's Day, if you've chosen that for an Indulgence day. It's another thing to sweet-talk your honey out of a five-pound *box* of chocolates, and nosh on them for a few days. Okay?

So pick and choose your Indulgences, and NEVER HAVE AN UNPLANNED INDULGENCE. If you're confronted with a carb food and you haven't planned an Indulgence, leave it alone!

Let me make another suggestion about Indulgences: Think hard to yourself about which carbohydrate foods *really* matter to you. For instance, in our traditional family Thanksgiving dinner, the carbohydrate foods include mashed potatoes, stuffing, candied sweet potatoes, creamed onions (flour in the cream sauce), gravy (again, flour as a thickener), cranberry sauce, banana-nut bread, oatmeal-molasses bread, pumpkin pie, and apple pie. Quite a list! But which of those foods do I *really* care about?

I couldn't care less about candied sweet potatoes, creamed onions, or banana-nut bread. Accordingly, I don't eat those things *at all*. Mashed potatoes are okay, I only have a little— maybe a spoonful.

But I *love* stuffing, especially with gravy, so I have a full-sized portion. I have half a slice or so of Mom's oatmeal-molasses bread, make sugar-free cranberry to go with my turkey, and I may have apple pie for dessert (although I make a *killer* low-carb pumpkin pie!). I eat only those carbs that are *truly desirable* to me. Your priorities will be different, but the process is the same: Decide which carb foods really matter to you, and eat *only* those carbs.

This is a good strategy in general: Why eat anything that's *not* what you want? For instance, since I hadn't had a dessert at that wedding on Memorial Day weekend, when I went to a terrific restaurant a couple of weeks later, I thought I might Indulge. But they had only fruit cobblers for dessert, and I really had my heart set on something chocolate. I passed on the Indulgence, so I still had one coming! I used my Indulgence instead to eat a big bag of Jalapeno Krunchers potato chips, the hottest and crunchiest potato chips on the planet. I think I enjoyed them more than I would have the desserts!

Another important thing to remember is that even at Indulgence meals, you *must* eat your *protein!* You are *never* excused from eating your protein. (Okay, if you have food poisoning or stomach flu, you're excused. But you won't be eating carbs, either!) For instance, on Christmas morning at my mom's house, I may eat a piece of her traditional coffee cake—but I also have a substantial serving of scrambled eggs and bacon. And at that Thanksgiving dinner we just passed, I also have plenty of turkey and low-carb vegetables like green beans, plus I'll have had my usual eggs for breakfast, so I'm not hitting the dinner table ravenous. Eating your protein will take the edge off your hunger for the carbs, limiting how much of them you're likely to eat. Also, the protein will help soften any blood sugar crash, with subsequent cravings, making it *much* easier to go right back to low carbing the next meal or the next day.

This picking and choosing what to have for your Indulgences leads me to another thought: Don't let other people buffalo you into eating something high carb that isn't what *you* want. Diet saboteurs are everywhere; some of them well meaning, some of them just plain malicious. They'll say things like, "Just a little taste won't hurt!" and "I made this just for you— you *have* to eat it!" But a little taste *can* hurt—it can unleash hunger and cravings, make you feel lousy and depressed, and add five pounds of water overnight. And unless you're a politician on the campaign trail, you don't *have* to eat anything you don't want to. Ever.

I've gotten to the point where I'm not even a *little* apologetic about this business of not eating stuff that's bad for me. No one else has to live with my fat, work through my mood and energy swings, pay my doctor bills, fight my cravings, or face my family history of heart disease and cancer. If people insist, I can get a little testy.

One relative is a case in point: A few years back, we were going to visit this relative around my birthday. She decided to cook me a birthday dinner; very nice—except she asked my husband what I could and could not eat, and after being told I didn't eat sugar or starch, proceeded to serve me potatoes and ice cream cake. She was *very* hurt and angry that I simply would *not* eat them. But why should I give in to that kind of emotional blackmail? She knew *in advance* that I didn't eat sugar or starch; I can only see serving them to me as a deliberate act. Don't give in to this kind of thing; Indulgences are far too precious to waste on what other people think you should eat.

If someone—usually a family member—is genuinely trying to sabotage your diet, repeatedly, it may call for either strong action or serious sneakiness. This happens far more often than you would believe! In particular, spouses often feel very threatened when their partner starts to change his or her eating habits and lose weight. They may feel pressured to change themselves, or they may feel that if their spouse becomes more attractive, they'll have more options and leave. Either way, it can get ugly. In a low-carb discussion on the Internet, a woman complained that her husband would deliberately open a box of chocolates and leave them next to her on the couch! Since this woman was not only dangerously obese, but also a diabetic, this was a very, very serious act. She chose to become sneaky: She'd keep a baggie in her pocket and slip a few chocolates into it so her husband would think she was eating them, then throw them away later.

Maybe you have that kind of willpower; many do not. Personally, faced with this situation, I would have asked *once,* nicely but firmly, that he stop trying to feed me candy. After that, the next time the box of chocolates appeared, I would have marched them to the bathroom and flushed them all down the toilet. After a few times of wasting his money on chocolates to feed the septic tank, I suspect that the husband would have given up. In this situation I also would have insisted on marriage counseling, to try to understand the insecurity and hostility that would drive a husband to treat his wife in a way that quite literally threatened her life.

Now and then there's a situation where you're faced with days and days of temptation. For instance, one friend went on a two-week cruise, with hot-and-cold running food and a fantastic dessert bar every night. In this situation, there are a few possibilities. One, you could decide that whatever program you've been doing up until then, for the interim you're on a Carb Controlling diet, and allow yourself to have that Indulgence once each day. If you're like me, you won't lose weight while doing this, but you shouldn't gain much, either. Another possibility would be to go on the Careful Carb Diet, and eat only plain super-premium ice cream from the dessert bar as one of your carb servings for the day.

What if you *really* screw up? What if you walk into the office one day, and there's a big box of Dunkin' Donuts on the table, and despite the fact that you didn't plan any kind of Indulgence—after all, Tuesday is hardly an occasion—you eat *three* of them. Now what?!

Well, first of all, *stop hating yourself!* This is not a moral issue here! I once had a low-carb cyberpal tell me she'd been "bad." I told her that unless she'd eaten the neighbor's child, she might have been unwise, but she hadn't been *bad*.

And don't bother playing little games with the scale! We all do this—moving it around on the floor, standing on the outsides of our feet, whatever. It doesn't change your true weight one iota, and you know it. You need to know the bad news—or the good news! Be honest with yourself; it's the path to success.

Next, go eat some protein! It will modify the crash and make it hurt less. And it *will* hurt, believe me!

Oh, I didn't warn you about that, did I? Yep, once you've been low carb for a few weeks, off the sugar, you'll find that you notice the druglike effects of the stuff. You'll feel lousy, and you'll have a hangover! You'll wonder how you ever ate so much of that stuff, and each time you do it, it will become less and less appealing.

Here's a quote from an e-mail I got from Tina, whom I taught to cut her carbs for energy—she titled the post "Walking Death!"

BLAH!!! I HAVE JUST MANAGED TO GET OFF MY COUCH FOR THE SECOND TIME IN 24 HOURS. I GOT HOME YESTERDAY AT 1:30 PM FROM PARTYING ON SATURDAY NIGHT AND HAVE BEEN LIKE WALKING DEATH EVER SINCE.

DANA, YOU DIDN'T WARN ME THAT AFTER HAVING NOT CONSUMED ENORMOUS AMOUNTS OF SUGAR THAT I WOULD GET ILL IF I DID CONSUME SUGAR AGAIN!

I'm not making that mistake with you. Consider yourself warned! Once you've given up sugar and other nasty, blood sugar wrecking carbs, you will feel anywhere from mildly hung-over to downright sick if you load up on them again. You'll also very likely find that the stuff just doesn't taste as good as you remembered. Most of the sweets I used to love now taste far, far too sweet to me, and I just can't eat them, even at an Indulgence. And *that*, my friend, is how you eventually learn not to miss sugar!

CHAPTER NINETEEN

Nutritional Supplements

L ET'S TALK ABOUT nutritional supplements. I should make it clear from the start that I am a person who believes in vitamins. I take a large number of vitamins, and have for a very long time. I am more and more convinced that they are worth the money, and then some. In fact, I consider them the best investment I've ever made.

Why can't we get all our vitamins and minerals from our food? A few hundred years ago, people probably could, and did, if they had access to good food. If you ate fresh free-range meat, lots of vegetables grown on composted soil, some seeds and nuts that you sprouted and didn't roast, and some fruit in season, you would probably get most of what you needed to deal with a world with little pollution.

However, that is hardly the case now. As long ago as the 1930s, the Congress officially stated that our soils were mineral depleted, and people who ate food grown on those soils would have mineral deficiencies. Minerals are lacking to begin with, and vitamins are lost in transit, on the shelf, or in the freezing or canning process, and during cooking.

Add to that the garbage in our air and water, and even such unquantified stressors as living under artificial light, and our dramatic reduction in exercise, and supplementation looks like a pretty good bet.

So what should you take? And, in particular, what can you take to help with your diet?

First of all, in my opinion EVERYONE should take a strong, full-spectrum multiple vitamin and mineral. Further, I feel that the highly advertised drugstore or grocery store multiple vitamins are close to worthless. First of all, they're not very well absorbed, and second, while they have okay doses of the vitamins they do include, they are missing some of the vitamins entirely and have very low doses of some minerals. Minerals, especially calcium and magnesium, take up a *lot* of room. Tablets that contain only calcium and magnesium usually require you to take three to six daily to get your RDA. If the necessary dose of just those two minerals won't fit in one tablet, think about all the vitamins and the other minerals you need and you'll see that a one-pill-a-day type supplement just isn't enough.

I would *strongly* recommend that you get a good, high-potency, three-to-six-tablet-, or capsule-a-day multiple vitamin with minerals that includes at least 100 percent of your RDA of calcium and magnesium. Alternatively, you can get a multiple vitamin that requires only one tablet a day, and also buy a good, broad-spectrum multiple mineral formula (just minerals), and take them together. Another possibility is the "pack vitamin"— little packets with four to six different tablets in them that you take every day. There are many good brands at health food stores, and many of the network marketing companies also have excellent formulas. What should you get for your money?

I would look for about 10,000 units of vitamin A. I know that beta carotene is very "in" right now, but I feel that fish liver oil A is excellent as well. I wouldn't buy a supplement that supplied less than 200 units of vitamin E, and feel that 400 units is better. Any supplement that is adequate in these, is likely to be adequate in vitamin D as well. If you find a supplement that includes vitamin K—which most people haven't even *heard* of— that's a clear sign the manufacturer is working to make it as complete as possible.

I would suggest that you buy a supplement that gives you good, big doses of all the B vitamins. Fifty units of each is great, but even 25 units is a healthy dose. (I say "units" here because some B vitamins are measured in milligrams (mg) while others are measured in micrograms (mcg). B vitamins should include thiamin (B1); riboflavin (B2); niacin or niacinamide (B3); pantothenic acid or pantothenate (B5); pyridoxine (B6); cobalamin or cyanocobalamin (B12); folic acid, sometimes called folate or folacin (this is an exception, by the way; a supplement should include 200 micrograms of folic acid); biotin; choline; and inositol. It's these last three that most often get left out. If you look for a supplement that includes choline and inositol, again, that's a sign that it's pretty complete.

B vitamins are water soluble, so you can't overdose. But you can get an imbalance, since supplementing one or two of them can cause your body to eliminate all of them faster. This happened back in the early 1980s, when it was publicized that B6 was a diuretic (would make you lose water). Women started taking truly frightening doses—as much as 1,000 milligrams of the stuff a day—of B6, without taking anything else. They, you should pardon the term, peed out all their other water-soluble vitamins and got good and sick. That's why I think it's best that you get your Bs from a good, complete multiple—you'll stay in balance.

Vitamin C is water-soluble, too. Did you know that human beings are one of a very, very few animals who don't make vitamin C in their bodies? Us and the other primates, guinea pigs, coho salmon, and some fruit bat somewhere, and that's about it. That's why your dog doesn't need vitamin C. Not only do most animals make their own vitamin C, but they make it in quantities far greater than the government recommends for human beings—the equivalent of an adult taking at least a few grams a day. I certainly would recommend that you take a minimum of 500 milligrams of vitamin C per day; I take far more—about 5,000 milligrams a day. If you smoke, you need more than a nonsmoker does—those 500 milligrams a day will just barely offset what you lose by smoking a pack a day, with none left over. (This is one of the reasons smokers age so fast!) If you're taking aspirin regularly, you'll need more, too.

It's easy to tell if you're getting more vitamin C than your body can use. If it's giving you gas and diarrhea, you're getting more than you need, and your body is throwing off the excess. If you're not getting these gastrointestinal symptoms, you're not getting too much. In fact, many nutritionists feel that you can best find your optimal dose of vitamin C by pushing your dose up until you start to get gas, and then backing it off just a bit. That's how I hit on a dose of 5,000 milligrams (5 grams) a day for my body. I've found, too, that when I get ill, I can take far, far more, as much as 25 grams a day, (25,000 milligrams) and never get gut trouble. Tells me my body is using all of it. As soon as I'm well, I have to drop back to 5 grams a day, or I'm running for the john!

Anyway, get at least 500 to 1,000 milligrams of vitamin C a day, okay?

Then there are the minerals. I'm not going to list every single mineral you should look for—most supplements that are adequate in the ones I do talk about will have the others, too. But there are a few minerals that everyone needs to be careful to get enough of, and a couple of minerals that are especially important to us low-carb dieters. I harp on minerals a lot, but I think they've been neglected—and I think they're truly vital, *especially* to dieters. Farmers know about a problem called "cribbing," when cattle start chewing on strange things like metal or rock. They know that if they give the cattle mineral supplements, the problem will go away. Well, in humans the same problem is known as pica, and it causes nearly uncontrollable cravings. Sometimes people eat really strange things like paint chips or dirt! I had one online low-carb buddy who had horrible sugar cravings every single day and absolutely hated vegetables—until she threw out her grocery store, one-pill-a-day supplement and bought a high-potency multivitamin and mineral from the health food store. Within a week, her cravings disappeared and lettuce started to taste okay to her. Pretty dramatic. *So get your minerals!*

First, as I mentioned before, make sure you're getting at least your RDA of **calcium**. The government has recently raised the RDA to one and a half grams, or 1,500 milligrams, a day. Since milk is quite high in carbohydrates—12 grams in one cup—you really can't drink the little-over-a-quart of milk a day you'd need to get your calcium. (Did you know it took that much? I know lots of people who drink a glass of milk a day and think they're covered.) There are some good low-carb sources of calcium— sardines (just about as good a food as you can get, if you like them), canned salmon, almonds, some of the dark green leafy vegetables like collards and turnip greens. Broccoli has more calcium in the leaves than in the stems and flowers, did you know that? Which means that if you buy frozen broccoli, you'll get a *little* more calcium in the cheaper chopped broccoli than in the more expensive broccoli spears because they put the leaves in the chopped kind.

Historically, people got a great deal of their calcium from *bones*. When people gnawed every last bit of meat off of a bone, they got a little of the bone, too. Calcium! (And the gristle is good for you, too; builds strong joints.) As we grew more civilized, bones were saved for making soup, and some of the calcium dissolved out of the bones into the broth, especially if some kind of acid, like vinegar or wine, was added. I save all my chicken bones in a bag in the freezer and make soup from them.

It's funny but true that the cutting edge in calcium supplements is something called hydroxyapatite, which is calcium in the form it appears in bones. Fifty years ago, nutrition pioneers, along with recommending a low-carbohydrate, high-protein diet, were recommending bone meal. I guess everything old really *is* new again!

Perhaps the greatest historical source of calcium was hard water, and even today, people who live where the water has a high content of calcium and magnesium live longer and have fewer health problems than people who live where the water is softer. If you have hard water in your neck of the woods, and it tastes okay, go ahead and drink it. It's good for you.

Most of us aren't willing to eat sardines every day, or make soup from bones, or eat enough broccoli leaves to get all our calcium, and we can't count on our tap water to contain enough. Yet calcium remains as vital as it ever was. Osteoporosis is no joke! Thousands of people die of the aftermath of hip fractures every year. Furthermore, calcium is needed for thousands of chemical reactions all over your body. Having too little can do everything from making your muscles tight and sore to raising your blood pressure to making it more likely you'll get cancer. Perhaps most important to the dieter, studies show that *people who get enough calcium are far more likely to reach their healthy weight than people who don't*. Take your supplements.

You should get at least half as much **magnesium** as you do calcium. Among other things, magnesium keeps calcium from forming stones in your kidneys. It also helps your body absorb and use the calcium. Too, magnesium is important for proper nerve function and can be calming, and who couldn't use that? Also, many people find that magnesium helps reduce carbohydrate cravings a *lot*. In particular, magnesium has a reputation for calming chocolate and sugar cravings. So that's at least a gram a day (1,500 milligrams) of calcium, and at least 750 milligrams of magnesium, right off the top.

Be careful about **iron;** it's possible to get too much, and if you're eating red meat, you're getting a fair amount in your diet. Excessive iron has been implicated in heart disease. Don't buy a supplement with more than the RDA of iron, and if you're eating red meat several times a week, you might look for one of the new, iron-free supplements. If you're a man or a pos menopausal woman, be aware that you're at a greater risk for iron overdose.

Be sure you're getting enough **iodine.** It's essential for thyroid function, and if your thyroid function is low, you'll have a very hard time losing weight. If you're not using iodized salt or eating fish several times a week, you might want to take kelp tablets—very inexpensive, a good source of iodine, and a good source of trace minerals in general. I take four to six a day, myself. Seaweed is a staple of Asian diets and very good for you—but not to my Western tastes!

Chromium is essential for carbohydrate metabolism, and a deficiency can destabilize blood sugar and cause sugar cravings. There is a lot of debate as to whether one form of chromium is better than another—the two most often recommended are GTF chromium (also called chromium polynicotinate) and chromium picolinate. Either GTF or picolinate should be okay, but make sure you're getting at least 200 micrograms a day, and 400 micrograms won't hurt you. **Zinc** seems to help chromium do its job, so be sure you're getting it, too. By the way, the classic sign of too little zinc in your body is white spots on your fingernails. Thirty to 60 milligrams of zinc is fine.

Vanadium, and especially a form called vanadyl sulfate, has been getting a lot of press lately because of its ability to fix insulin resistance to some degree. Twenty-five micrograms should be plenty.

Chromium picolinate and vanadyl sulfate have been touted recently as "super fat burners." I consider this a *huge* exaggeration. However, I do think they can strengthen your carbohydrate metabolism and help your diet a lot. Further, taking these two minerals over the months that you're actively losing may mean that when the time comes for maintenance, you can afford a few more grams of carb a day than you would otherwise. Anything that allows you 60 or 70 grams a day of carb, instead of 30 or 40, is worth taking!

By the way, you want to seek out the minerals that are "chelated"—which means they're bound to a protein to help them cross the intestinal lining and be absorbed. These will say "chelated" or "chelate" on the label. Chelated minerals are VASTLY superior to cheap mineral supplements, which are little more than ground rock.

As I mentioned earlier, some of the top-of-the-line supplements are now using a form of calcium called hydroxyapatite. This is the form calcium takes in your bones and is very absorbable—it's naturally protein-bound. I take a hydroxy-apatite-type calcium supplement myself.

Let me remind you again of a mineral I mentioned back in the section about the Basic Low-Carb Diet—**potassium.** If you were feeling really good on a very low-carb diet, and then all of a sudden feel tired and wrung out and weak and achy, you may need a potassium supplement. Because of the fast water loss in the first few weeks, and because a low-fat/high-carb diet encourages your body to throw off potassium at the same time it causes sodium retention, many people take a little while to balance out the sodium/potassium thing. You can add two or three potassium pills through the day—they're pretty low dosage—or you can buy Morton's Lite Salt, which is about half potassium chloride and tastes okay. Multiple vitamins do not contain appreciable amounts of potassium.

When you find a multiple vitamin and mineral formula, or a multiple vitamin with minerals plus a multiple mineral formula, that gives you all these things—enough A and E; plenty of C; *all* the Bs in ample doses; all of the calcium, magnesium, zinc, chromium, and vanadium you need, in well-absorbed chelate form—you can feel confident that it will be adequate in other nutrients—manganese, copper, zinc, selenium, etc.—as well.

Other supplements you should know about: If you're feeling a bit constipated, you may certainly take **fiber supplements** on a low-carb diet. FiberCon tablets are fine, as is sugar-free Metamucil, or any fiber product that has no sugar in it. READ YOUR LABELS! Probably your best choice for extra fiber is, as mentioned earlier, **flax seed.** If you're eating plenty of low-carb vegetables, constipation shouldn't be a problem, but if you're having trouble warming up to lots of salad and broccoli, you may well need some help. Also keep in mind that magnesium deficiency can cause constipation—you've heard of Milk of Magnesia as a laxative, right? If you're having trouble with constipation, make sure you're getting your magnesium.

I personally have had good results with one of the newest "wonder supplements," **DHEA.** DHEA is a hormone precursor; that is, a substance your body uses to make a whole bunch of different hormones, including estrogen and testosterone. Levels are naturally high in your twenties, and then decline after age thirty. DHEA supplementation in lab animals caused them to lose fat and gain muscle and have fewer heart problems, more energy, and a higher sex drive. It's had about the same effect on me—within three days of starting to take DHEA, I found myself dancing in the kitchen, I had so much extra energy, and I lost seven pounds in the first week or so that I was on it.

Youngsters don't need DHEA—I wouldn't recommend it much before age thirty-five—and I would stick with what are called "replacement dosages," which is to say just enough to approximate youthful levels. That would be from 5 to 50 milligrams a day. (I take 12 milligrams per day. I tried taking more, but I got "teenaged" acne!) Bodybuilders are using DHEA in *huge* doses as a steroid replacement, and it seems to work well, but I wonder about the safety of increasing hormone levels that dramatically for long periods of time. You should know that DHEA is controversial—please be cautious. You may want to consult your doctor.

I also take another hormone precursor called **pregnenolone**. Pregnenolone can be differentiated into a wider variety of hormones than DHEA. Indeed, your body can make DHEA and all its resultant hormones from pregnenolone. But it can also make progesterone, the other female hormone, from pregnenolone, which it cannot do from DHEA. I have read a fair amount about the disadvantages of estrogen "unopposed" by progesterone, and suspect that pregnenolone may be better, especially for women, for this one reason alone. Pregnenolone seems to have mood-elevating and memory-enhancing properties that DHEA lacks. Too, pregnenolone was widely used as a safe, effective treatment for arthritis before steroid drugs were invented.

Bottom line, I would strongly recommend that you take a high-potency multiple, with plenty of chelated calcium and magnesium, at least 200 micrograms of GTF chromium or chromium picolinate, and 25 micrograms of vanadium or vanadyl sulfate. Even better would be a product with a broad spectrum of chelated minerals. Make sure you're getting enough iodine. For trace minerals, you can take one of the colloidal mineral supplements that are on the market, or the newly popular coral calcium. Or you can do as I do and take kelp tablets and use unrefined sea salt, both good sources of trace minerals.

If you want to maximize your good eicosanoids, adding an EPA and a GLA supplement couldn't hurt. And I personally swear by DHEA and pregnenolone, but they're controversial enough that I'd recommend that you do a little research on your own before you decide they're right for you. *The Super Hormone Promise,* by Dr. William Regelson, is a good place to start.

CHAPTER TWENTY

Low-Carb Specialty Products

W HEN I WENT low carb in 1995, there were virtually no low-carb specialty products. After all, nobody ate this way! Everybody knew that a low-fat diet high in grains and beans was the path to slimness, health, and energy. Robert Atkins was that guy who had written that fad diet book back in the 1970s that everyone knew was discredited now. Make special products for low-carbohydrate dieters? Hah! Bring on the Snackwells and Lean Cuisine!

As a result, a low-carbohydrate diet—as I mentioned in the first chapter—virtually *forced* you to eat real, fresh, unprocessed foods. All we had were meat, fish, poultry, eggs, cheese, and butter, oils, nuts and seeds, low-carb vegetables, and low-sugar fruits.

What a difference eight years can make! Low-carbohydrate dieting has not only been vindicated by medical research, it is the rage. Millions upon millions of people, seeing their friends and relatives go on "that crazy diet" only to lose weight and find good health, have joined us. All of this means that we are now a *market*. And America is *nothing* if it is not market-driven.

Accordingly, there are now something like a zillion new low-carb products on the market. As with all classes of products, some of the low-carb products are quite good, some are truly god-awful, and still others are somewhere in between.

However, all low-carb specialty products I've run across have one thing in common: They're all expensive; certainly more expensive than their high-carb counterparts.

Don't get me wrong, I'm not saying that these products are overpriced. They're not. They're expensive because they are, indeed, *specialty* products, mostly made by small companies, in smallish batches, for a specialty market. They're also more expensive because they are made with higher-quality ingredients. Refined white flour, corn syrup, sugar, cornstarch, etc., are *cheap*, which is why they're so widely used. Replace those cheap commodities with things like protein powder, ground nuts, and low-carbohydrate sweeteners, and the nutritional value of these foods skyrockets—but so does the cost. You know that macaroni and cheese you buy for thirty cents a box? The same-size box of low-carb macaroni and cheese will set you back between four and five dollars.

You see how this could run up the food bill a tad.

And this is one of my *major* concerns about low-carb specialty foods: They are so expensive that people who get into the habit of using them regularly get fed up with the strain on the budget. They decide that they can't afford to eat low carb, and quit. This is foolish, both because there's absolutely no reason why you *have* to buy any low-carb specialty stuff—you'll do just fine on grocery store food—and because few things are more expensive than ill health. Still, this happens, and I do hear frequent complaints about how expensive low carbing is.

Please avoid this trap. Low-carb specialty foods are useful for providing a welcome variety to our menus, for making the transition to this way of eating, and for dealing with cravings, but they should *not* become a mainstay of your diet. Do not try to make your low-carb diet resemble your old, Standard American Diet. That's the diet that got you in trouble in the first place, remember? The basis of your diet should be the foods I mentioned above: meat, fish, poultry, eggs, cheese, butter and oil, nuts and seeds, low-carbohydrate vegetables, and low-sugar fruits.

This is true not only because low-carb specialty products are expensive, but also because many of them are highly processed foods that simply do *not* offer the same nutritional value of unprocess-ed, natural foods, and also because most of these low-carb foods, although lower in carbohydrate than the foods they replace, are not as low in carbohydrate as animal protein foods.

So use these foods, if you like, and be glad we have them, but keep them in perspective—an occasional treat, not staples of your diet, okay?

With that understood, let's talk a little about what's out there.

Artificial Sweeteners

People sometimes give me a hard time about artificial sweeteners. "How can you recommend something artificial?" they demand. "After all, at least sugar is natural." Yeah. So is rattlesnake venom. So are death angel mushrooms. So is tobacco. Natural is no guarantee of safety.

That being said, I do not mean to suggest that artificial sweeteners are 100 percent safe. I know of *nothing* that is 100 percent safe. The question is not, "Are artificial sweeteners completely safe?" The question is, "Are artificial sweeteners *safer than what they replace?*" And to this I believe the answer is a resounding *yes*.

Still, I hope that you will not eat and/or drink artificially sweetened foods and beverages in the same quantity that most Americans eat their sugary counterparts. The ideal is to slowly back away from feeling that every day requires some concentrated sweet-flavored food, and to return sweets to their rightful place, as occasional treats for special occasions. Once the sweet flavor comes without the blood sugar rush and resulting crash, and the physical addiction is broken, this becomes easier to do.

However, if at first, having a sugar-free dessert a few times a week, or even once a day, is what it takes to keep you on your low-carbohydrate program, I think that beats the heck out of giving up! I know that I had sugar-free chocolate mousse in the refrigerator most of the time for the first few months after I took the low-carb plunge.

I'm assuming that you already know about saccharine and

aspartame, most commonly known as Sweet'N Low (saccharine) and Equal (aspartame). You may not be aware of the newest artificial sweetener, called sucralose—trade name Splenda. But you will. You will.

Sucralose was approved in the United States a couple of years ago, after being used in other countries for several years. It's an artificial sweetener that is actually *made from sugar.* Scientists somehow patched in some extra chlorine and came up with a molecule that the body doesn't recognize—and therefore passes through.

For some strange reason, the extra chlorine makes sucralose *600 times sweeter than sugar.* In order to make it easier to use, sucralose is "bulked"—mixed with something less sweet. To make the table sweetener Splenda, the sucralose is bulked with maltodextrin. This makes Splenda the same sweetness as sugar, so it's easy to know how much to use.

Unfortunately, maltodextrin also adds carbohydrate. Splenda has 0.5 grams of carbohydrate per teaspoon, or 24 grams of carbohydrate per cup. This is only one-eighth the carbohydrate of sugar, but is not inconsiderable when using Splenda in recipes. Many low carbers are hoping that MacNeil—the company that makes Splenda—will release liquid Splenda in the United States. Liquid Splenda is carb-free and is available in some other countries (and to food processors, who use it in things like diet soda). No explanation yet why MacNeil won't release it here! In the meanwhile, we'll just have to count those maltodextrin carbs.

If you think you don't like the taste of artificial sweeteners, you *have* to try Splenda. It tastes really good—no bitter aftertaste, no weird chemical "off" flavor. Further, it stands up to heat, so you can cook with it in ways you never could cook with Equal. Keep in mind, however, that Splenda only provides sweetness—it does not crystalize or brown like sugar, nor does it hold moisture in baked goods the way that sugar does. Still, Splenda is a *huge* step forward for artificial sweeteners. If you haven't tried it, you should.

Polyols or Sugar Alcohols

Polyols, also known as sugar alcohols, are a class of sweeteners widely used in commercially produced sugar-free candy, baked goods, and ice cream. There are several polyols, and most of their names end with "ol"—maltitol, lactitol, sorbitol, mannitol, xylitol, and the like. (There's also one called isomalt. I don't know why.)

Polyols *are* carbohydrates. However, they are carbohydrates with very big molecules—so big that it is difficult for the human body to digest or absorb them. This means that for most people, polyols apparently cause far less of a rise in blood sugar and less of an insulin release than sugar.

However, this is somewhat controversial. There are low-carb dieters who shun polyols as carbs, and there are others who embrace them with a somewhat unhealthy fervor. Some dieters say these products throw them out of ketosis, other say that—in moderation—they don't. This is apparently because different polyols are absorbed to different degrees, and are even absorbed differently by different people—very much a "your mileage may vary" issue.

Polyols also have another drawback: Like all indigestible carbohydrates—think fiber—they can cause gas and diarrhea if eaten to excess. What's "excess"? Ah, there's the rub. Again, this varies from person to person. Some people find that even *one piece* of polyol-based candy is enough to cause a bad case of the runs, complete with painful gut cramps. Other people find that so long as they eat these products with restraint—no more than, say, one candy bar a day—they have no problems. The only way to find out is experimentation, I'm afraid. Be smart, and *go easy!*

So why, with these drawbacks, are polyols used at all? Why not just use Splenda or aspartame or something?

Because unlike those completely uncarbohydrate-like sweeteners, the polyols can give all of the textures that sugar gives, along with the desired sweetness. The good polyol sweetened products are *virtually indistinguishable* from their sugary counterparts. Marshmallows are spongy and gooey. Gummy worms are—well, gummy. Caramel is soft and chewy. Chocolate melts in your mouth. Brownies are rich and fudgy. Ice cream is creamy and soft. These are textures that are impossible to get with artificial sweeteners. You can see, then, the appeal of the polyol-sweetened products.

All I can say is *be careful*. Pay attention to what these products do to your hunger and your cravings and your weight. If you cannot eat polyol-sweetened foods in moderation, it is very much best not to eat them at all. And always remember that regardless of what these products do to your weight loss and addiction triggers, overindulgence is likely to be disastrous to your gut—not to mention your social life.

If you are diabetic, it is *vital* that you monitor your blood sugar after eating polyol-sweetened products. It is also important to remember that these products often have sources of carbohydrate other than the polyols—for instance, no-sugar-added ice cream still has the carbohydrate that comes from the milk it's made with. *These are not "free" foods by any means.*

They are also not particularly nutritious foods. A sugar-free candy bar or brownie is *never* a substitute for a chicken Caesar salad for lunch. Got it? For those who can tolerate them, these are fun fringe foods, nothing more.

Two more useful things to know about polyols:

Sugar-free cough drops are made with polyols, usually sorbitol. These sure beat the sugary kind if you have a hacking cough.

Sugar-free stuff that's aimed at the low-carb market will often have the polyols left out of the carbohydrate count. You'll know this is the case if your candy bar says something like, "Only 2 grams of effective carb per bar!" on the label. However, *most sugar-free candy is made with polyols.* This means that if you're in a candy store—Fanny May, See's, Fanny Farmer, whatever they have in your neck of the woods—the sugar-free candy is probably polyol sweetened, and probably has an effective carb count similar to the "low-carb specialty" candies, even though the labeling will say it has more carbs. Do watch out. Sometimes "sugar-free" stuff is sweetened with honey, fructose, or concentrated fruit juice, all of which are most definitely SUGAR. But if you can't get the low-carb specialty brands near you, your local candy store may have sugar-free candy that will work for you—again, *in moderation*.

So What Low-Carb Products Are Out There?

Here's a quick rundown of some of the low-carb specialty products available today:

- *Breads and bagels:* These are often quite good, but keep an eagle eye on the portion size listed on the label. I've seen low-carb bagels with a label claiming only 4 grams a serving—but a serving was only one-third of a bagel!

- *Tortillas:* Useful not only for eating with fajitas and burritos and for making quesadillas, but also in place of Chinese mu shu pancakes. I've even heard of people using them in place of lasagna noodles! Be aware that low-carb tortillas, while tasty, are not identical to either flour or corn tortillas in flavor or texture.

- *Jams, jellies, and condiments:* These do contain the carbohydrate from whatever fruit or vegetable was used to make them, but not added sugars. Generally very good in quality, especially Jok'n Al brand, imported from New Zealand.

- *Sugar-free coffee-flavoring syrups:* I know of two widely distributed brands: Da Vinci and Atkins, with Da Vinci usually being easier to find. Your best bet to find these is to look in a gourmet coffee shop, the sort that sells all kinds of flavored coffees. Sugar-free coffee-flavoring syrup comes in vanilla, chocolate, hazelnut, and a range of other flavors. Another nice use for these is to put a couple of tablespoonfuls in a tall glass, add half a cup of cream, and fill with chilled sparkling water.

- *Pastas:* I have yet to find a brand of low-carb pasta that has really impressed me, but some of it is sort of okay. I find that the texture of the pastas is off—they cook up either too soft or too chewy. Still, the stuff sells like low-carb hotcakes, so somebody must really like it. If you are having a hard time passing up pasta, these products are worth a try.

- *Cold cereals:* I've tried three low-carb cold cereals. One, called *Keto Crisp,* is quite similar to Rice Krispies in texture and flavor. This is now available in a chocolate flavor as well. The second is called *Nuttlettes,* and is very much like Grape Nuts. These are both quite good if you're fond of the cereals they imitate. Both of these "cereals" are made from soy, which some people think is a lifesaving wonder food, and others of us—myself included—aren't sure is safe in large quantities. It's a moot point for me, since I just don't miss Rice Krispies or Grape Nuts enough to bother with these cereals. (Although *Keto Crisp* makes a mean cookie bar!) However, if you do miss cold cereal, these products are quite good and quite low in carbohydrate and high in protein.

  The third low-carb "cereal" I've tried is by Gram's Gourmet, and is sold both as a granola and a snack. Called Flax 'n' Nut Crunchies, this is a product I would definitely buy again. Made mostly of nuts and seeds, and both in sweet, granolalike flavors such as Vanilla Almond and Cinnamon and in savory flavors like Cheese, Flax 'n' Nut Crunchies have plenty of protein and healthy fats to keep you satisfied through a morning's work, and has less than 5 grams of usable carb per serving. It also has no polyols, so even those who are polyol sensitive can enjoy it. It does have a modest quantity of soy, but not a lot. Not exactly like grain-based granola, but good stuff, and not a highly processed food.

  However, low-carb cold "cereals" are hitting the market at a quick pace, and I know there are several I haven't tried. Keep your eyes open!

- *Hot cereal:* There are a few low-carb hot "cereals" on the market at this writing, and I've heard good reviews on them. The one I've tried is Cream of Flax, from Gram's Gourmet, and I like it very much. Hot flax cereal is a great way to get the EPAs and soluble fiber that flax has to offer. There's also a low-carb "grits extender" on the market, for all you southerners!

- *Protein chips:* These are okay, but not so wonderful that I've bothered to buy them often. Of the "regular" chips, these most resemble tortilla chips, but the texture is noticeably different. If you're mad for a bag of chips, these are worth a try, at any rate. Me, I'd rather have pumpkin seeds.
- *Protein meal replacement shakes:* Mostly quite good, and certainly useful for folks who can't face cooked food first thing in the morning or who need a fast, take-along lunch. Available in a wide range of flavors.
- *Protein bars:* These seem to be everywhere these days. Protein bars range from pretty darned good to absolutely wretched, sometimes within the same brand. You'll have to try a few to see which ones you like. Be aware that there is a lot of controversy about low-carb protein bars. Virtually all of them contain glycerine, to make them moist and chewy—the controversy is over whether or not glycerine acts like a carbohydrate in some ways in the body. Many people find that these bars knock them out of ketosis, while others don't have a problem. Pay attention to your body! Also be aware that Twin Lab puts out a Metabolift bar that includes ephedrine, which may or may not be what you want. Read your labels!
- *Low-carb baking mixes:* These are proliferating like crazy; Atkins, in particular, is putting out a bunch of them. Keto brand makes several, too. You can buy everything from plain "low-carb bake mix," which replaces things like Bisquick, to low-carb brownie mix, pancake mix, cookie mix, corn bread mix, and even bread machine mixes to make yeast breads of various types. Quality varies—for instance, I liked the Atkins brownie mix just fine but wasn't crazy about their corn bread mix—but the economics don't. All of these things are pretty steep. The sweet mixes tend to use polyols.
- *Cookies and brownies:* Getting better every day, and many quite good. I've had low-carb brownies that were superb, and some very nice oatmeal cookies, as well. Nearly all have polyols.

- *Crackers:* Along with fiber crackers, I've had some low-carb, high-protein crackers that were quite good. Worth looking out for.
- *Psyllie Snacks:* I know these sound strange, but this chip-like snack made from psyllium fiber—the same fiber used in Metamucil—is remarkably good. Remember that they're fiber, and go easy!
- *Muffins:* Some quite good, others not so brilliant, and often the same brand is good or bad, depending on which flavor you choose. You'll just have to try them and see which you like. Some have polyols, some don't.
- *Other sweet low-carb baked goods:* I've tried commercially made low-carb cheesecake and cake rolls. The cheesecake was pretty good, but I can make better for far less money. I didn't like the cake rolls at all—I found them overwhelmingly sweet—but know that they sell quite well, so *somebody* must like them. Some have polyols, some don't.
- *Chocolate bars and other chocolate candy:* These, my friend, are generally *superb*. The best of the low-carb chocolate candy—Carbolite, Pure De-Lite, Ross, Darrell Lea, Low Carb Chef—is *indistinguishable* from its sugar-laden counterparts. You can get low-carb chocolate in both milk and dark. There are peanut butter cups, crispy bars, turtles, you name it. I haven't had a really bad sugar-free chocolate yet. All sweetened with polyols, so eat in moderation! There are one or two brands that include hydrogenated vegetable oils, which are very definitely not recommended.
- *Other sugar-free candies:* You can, if you look, find sugar-free taffies, hard candies, marshmallows, jellybeans, all manner of things. Again, the quality of these tends to be excellent. The *bulk* of these candies is made up of polyols, so go *very* easy—I've known utter disaster to follow the consumption of a dozen taffies!
- *No-sugar-added ice cream:* This stuff is not officially sugar-free, since the milk it's made from contains lactose, a sugar. It is, however, much lower in sugar and usable carbs than

regular ice cream. Breyer's makes this, and so does the company called Edy's in the eastern part of the country, and Dreyer's in the west. Even the folks at Healthy Choice are jumping on the bandwagon and putting out a no-sugar variety. Edy's is the brand I've had, and god help me, it's *too* good. I can't buy it often, because it triggers *seriously* addictive and compulsive behavior. Approach with caution, and *do not sit down with the carton and a spoon.* The Voice of Experience, here. The no-sugar-added ice creams generally use a combination of sweeteners, including aspartame and polyols, and sometimes others. There are also sugar-free ice pops and fudge pops available; these generally do not have polyols. Good if you like that sort of thing.

Starch Blockers

What exactly are starch blockers? Do they work?!

Starch blockers (also called "carb cutters") are an extract of a bean called *Phaseolus vulgaris;* the extract is properly called phaseolamin. This substance, phaseolamin, is said to neutralize the enzyme responsible for digesting starches, thus allowing a certain amount of any given starch food to pass through your system undigested and unabsorbed. This process does, indeed, work in a test tube ("in vitro"). The big question was whether it actually works in your body ("in vivo").

Why wouldn't it work in your body if it works in a test tube? For the simple reason that the phaseolamin itself is a protein. Proteins are digested in your stomach. Starches, on the other hand, are digested in your small intestine. If the phaseolamin is digested in the stomach, there theoretically will be none left to neutralize the enzyme in your intestine. Result? No starch blocking.

On the other hand, I was around when starch blockers first hit the market back in the early 1980s—I was working in the health food industry at the time. And I did see a few people who claimed to be getting good weight loss results with them. Further, the story going around was that this substance had been discovered when some farmers started feeding their cattle raw

Phaseolus vulgaris beans and the cattle started losing weight—
which could mean that raw beans aren't any better food for
cattle than they are for humans, but also suggested that the idea
might actually work.

How to find out? Here's what I did:

First of all, I had some starch blockers on hand that had been
sent to me to review. So that was taken care of. Next, I went out
and bought an inexpensive glucose meter and test strips.

Then I decided on a couple of foods to test. I knew I didn't
want to test really nasty, high-impact carbs like white bread or
cold cereal—too hard on the body, and anyway, they just didn't
appeal to me. I settled on brown rice and 100 percent whole
grain rye bread as my test foods. These also had the advantage of
being easy to measure, to make sure I ate pretty darned close to
the same quantity for each test. Brown rice I could measure carefully before and after cooking, and the rye bread comes in a nice,
neat, brick-shaped loaf—once I had it sliced on the bread slicer at
the health food store, the slices were quite uniform in size.

So I was set to go. I got up one morning and took my fasting blood sugar. I then ate a carefully measured portion of
brown rice, and proceeded to take my blood sugar reading every
fifteen to twenty minutes for the next couple of hours. (I trust
you realize that this means that I had to stick *lots* of little holes
in my pinkies. Don't say I never do anything for you.)

I then did the same thing, but took a starch blocker capsule
first, about seven minutes before I began eating.

I repeated the experiment, but this time I used two slices of
100 percent whole grain rye bread as my serving of starch,
instead of brown rice.

I repeated the experiment several times. I tried it with two or
three starch blockers. I tried it taking the starch blockers *just* as
I started eating, or taking them halfway through eating, or taking one just before starting to eat, one halfway through, and one
just as I finished. (It had been suggested to me that perhaps more
of the phaseolamin would make it past the stomach and into the
intestine if the starch blocker were taken *with* the starch food,

rather than several minutes ahead of time. This interested me, since the package directions on most of these products recommend taking starch blockers five to ten minutes before eating the starch food.)

"So," you're thinking, "what were the **RESULTS! C'MON!** Spit it out!" Oh, okay.

Does phaseolamin work? My scientific opinion is, "Kinda."

I clearly was still absorbing carbohydrates when I took the starch blocker, no matter how much I took—the most I took with one serving of carb food was four starch blocker capsules. My blood sugar did go up, and fairly sharply. I still got a blood sugar drop *in some cases* that was steep enough to make me hungry. However, when I took three starch blockers, and took them with and after eating the food, something very interesting happened: My blood sugar went up pretty high, but it *came down more slowly.* Something seemed to be moderating the blood sugar crash, so that even three hours later, my blood sugar had not dropped back to the original fasting level. I do not have even a working hypothesis why this should be so, but it happened more than once, so I'm thinking it's not an anomaly.

Also, in *most* cases, my blood sugar did not go up *quite* as far when I took the starch blockers as when I did not—in general, it topped out about twenty points lower than it did without the starch blockers, although there was one exception—but then, exactly *when* you draw blood makes a big difference, and I'd probably have to repeat these experiments until my poor little pinkies fell off to get really seriously conclusive data. Still, I can draw a few conclusions:

- Do not figure that starch blockers are a way to get out of eating a low-carb diet. These pills do not work so well that you can simply swallow them and keep on eating all the French fries and bread and chips and cereal you want, while losing weight and getting the health benefits of reduced insulin levels. They are not a magic bullet. If you're carb intolerant, you'll still need to avoid these foods for the most part. Trying to "change without changing" is not a useful strategy, it's a dangerous fantasy.

- Starch blockers may, however, help mitigate some of the effects of an occasional Indulgence. They will not completely protect you from the effects—or, at least, they don't completely protect me from the effects—but they may help moderate the blood sugar roller coaster. This may mean that you don't gain quite as much, and just as important, may keep the subsequent blood sugar crash, hunger, and cravings to a minimum, making it easier to go right back on the straight and narrow.

- Starch blockers may also be an okay strategy for cutting back even further on some of the carbs in some of the carb-reduced specialty products out there. For instance, if you're going to eat, say, half a low-carb bagel, you're still looking at 6 or 8 grams of usable carb. You may be able to knock off a few of those by taking starch blockers.

- If you're planning to use starch blockers with regular, non-reduced-carb foods, take two or three of them, not just the one capsule that the label says will block 400 grams of starch. It won't; you need to take enough that some of the phaseolamin makes it past your stomach undigested.

- Do take starch blockers with the food, rather than five to ten minutes before. Indeed, taking one or two just as you start eating, and another halfway through or even when you're finished, seems to help a bit.

- Keep in mind that undigested carbs in your gut can cause gas or even diarrhea. I wouldn't use these on a big date, no matter how tempting the restaurant you're going to.

- These things are expensive. Unless you've got big bucks, the price and the need to use more than one capsule will probably limit your use to the occasional Indulgence.

- Remember that these things do not work at all on sugar. Not even a tiny bit. Only on starch. You have been warned.

One more thought: If you're considering getting some starch blockers—and again, while I think they're seriously overhyped, they seem to have their uses—I'd suggest a quick prayer to God or Destiny or whatever you believe in, thanking Him, Her, or it that you're so very wealthy that you can afford to buy expensive pills so that you won't digest and absorb the food you eat!

CHAPTER TWENTY-ONE

Plateaus

OH, THE DREADED plateau! Also known as frustration squared. Not part of just low-carb dieting; everybody who's ever been on any kind of weight loss diet has hit a plateau from time to time. Low carbers are no different. Plateaus are discouraging, no question about it. When you're being "good," it's almost more than a body can bear to have your weight loss stall for a few weeks, or even a few months.

So what to do?

Well, first, take a mental inventory of any other benefits you've noticed from your low-carb diet: improved energy, better blood work, reduced allergies, less hunger, clearer mind, better moods, whatever. These, for me, were the biggest reason I never seriously considered quitting during my plateaus, some of which lasted waaaay too long, for my liking! I was unwilling to gain back what I had lost, or to go back to feeling tired and logy and hungry, so I stuck it out.

Second, get very honest with yourself and make sure you've really been sticking to whichever program you've chosen. If you're on the Basic Low-Carb diet, get out the food count book and count your carb grams for a week, to be sure you're not getting more than you think you are. Remember that food labels allow manufacturers to fudge a bit, so count foods that say "0 grams per serving" as 0.5 grams, and foods that say "less than

1 gram per serving" as 1 gram. And if you haven't been vigilant about reading labels, start! If you've been on a Carb Controlling plan, be sure you haven't been stretching that hour for the Reward Meal. In other words, be sure that you're really plateaued, rather than cheating.

If you're sure you're not slipping on the diet, and a plateau lasts more than a few weeks, it may be time to try changing something. What? There are a whole lot of adjustments you can make, and different changes help different people.

Your Mileage May Vary

That's the phrase we use on the Internet to summarize the concept that different things have different effects on different people. All of the things in this section have a very large effect on some people, and a much lesser effect—or no perceptible effect—on others.

First of all, with this book in hand, you're well prepared to try a different approach to low carbing. So do it! If you've been doing the Carb Controlling Diet, try the Careful Carb program, or go to a Basic Low-Carb diet. If you've been doing the Basic Low-Carb plan, eating three meals a day, try it eating six smaller meals, or try a day or two of carbing up. If you've been eating a whole lot of extra protein and not a lot of fat, try eating more healthy fats and only your minimum allowance of protein. If you've been eating just the minimum of protein and a lot of fat, try switching that. You get the picture.

But change only one thing at a time, okay? Otherwise you may never know what worked. And remember that your body is a remarkable thing and can adapt to almost anything; throwing it a curve now and then can be a good idea.

Here, in no particular order, are some things that affect some people's weight loss a lot, and others not at all.

- *Eat the same quantity of food, but divide it up into smaller, more frequent feedings.* This alone has, in some instances, been enough to cause weight loss.
- *Drop dairy.* Yep, it's hard—dairy is versatile and yummy—but I've known a fair number of people for whom this was

the thing that did the trick. If you do this, up your calcium
supplements.

- *Axe the aspartame.* Roughly half of low-carb dieters find
  that artificially sweetened beverages interfere with their
  ability to lose weight, or will act as a "trigger"—something
  that makes them hungry. Why this should be is a matter of
  controversy. Some—Dr. Robert Atkins among them—say
  that aspartame (NutraSweet, Equal) has a negative effect
  on your body's ability to burn fat. Dr. Atkins used to allow
  aspartame; you'll find it in his book. Since then he has
  stated, in his newsletter, that he feels that aspartame is dan
  gerous, and that it interferes with fat burning on a chemical
  level.

Others state that some people are so hypersensitive to carbohydrates that even the *taste* of sweetness will cause an insulin
surge. The Hellers, in particular, claim this. Still others say this
has never been demonstrated in clinical tests.

Still another camp feels that the aspartame is not the problem; that instead the problem is citric acid, widely used in beverages and other processed foods. Apparently citric acid can
interfere with ketosis, that state of rapid fat burning. Citric acid
shows up in most diet beverages—sodas and other beverages
such as Crystal Light and diet iced tea mix, and even unsweetened, unflavored bottled iced tea. Some iced tea at fast-food
joints has citric acid, too—if you've ever gotten iced tea that had
a strange, sour undertaste, that was citric acid. It also can be an
ingredient in sugar-free gelatin desserts.

If you're having trouble losing, or you're still hungry and
craving, on your low-carb program, and you're certain you've
been good about cutting out the carbs, try cutting down on, or
cutting out, the artificially sweetened beverages. Drink iced tea
sweetened, if you need it, with saccharine (Sweet'n Low) or stevia,
the natural sweetener I mentioned in the diet shake section.

- *Cut out the treats.* If you've been eating a lot of low-carb
  specialty products—pastas, crackers, cookies, candy, etc.
  —you may be getting more stray carbs than you think.

Remember that the labels on these products often do their best to minimize the carb content by subtracting out any "inactive" carbs, like polyols, and starches with a low blood sugar impact. Yet there's reason to suspect that these ingredients *do* cause at least some insulin release and refilling of glycogen stores. Go back to meat, poultry, fish, eggs, cheese, nuts, seeds, and vegetables for a few weeks and see what happens.

- Adjust your fat-to-protein ratio. Wouldn't you know it, level of fat intake is controversial even in low-carb circles! Some, like Dr. Robert Atkins, Dr. Herman Taller, and Dr. Richard MacKarness, feel that more fat is better; that fat suppresses appetite, deepens ketosis, stimulates fat burning. Dr. Taller in his 1962 book recommended that his readers drink an ounce of safflower oil before every meal! MacKarness actually named his 1958 low-carb book *Eat Fat & Grow Slim*. And Dr. Atkins, one of my heroes, recommended eating plenty of fat, especially in the first few weeks, because it encourages ketosis. He even outlined a "Fat Fast" for those who have a great deal of trouble losing—1,000 calories a day, 900 of which are pure fat! He felt that the Fat Fast is the quickest way to burn fat, faster than eating nothing at all. Not much fun, though, unless you're awfully fond of macadamia nuts and cream cheese.

Others are more moderate. The Eadeses don't want you to *avoid* fat, but they don't push it, either. And the Hellers give instructions on how to make their program both carb controlled and low fat if you want to, though they don't specifically recommend this.

I have known low-carb dieters who have added extra fat to their diets and improved their weight loss. I also have known low-carb dieters who cut *back* a bit on fat and improved their weight loss! Talk about "your mileage may vary"! All I can suggest is experimentation.

One thing I'm pretty sure of: The more you are willing to do without carbs, the more fat you can afford to eat. On the other hand, a low-fat/high-carb diet has been disastrous, overall, to the health of the nation! So don't decide to eat protein, low-impact carbs, and no fat. *Bad* idea. Even Ann Louise Gittleman, former nutrition director at The Pritikin Center, has now stated that good fats are essential for health *and* for fat burning. Don't let your fat intake drop an inch below 30 percent of your calories.

Also be aware that there are specific fats that stimulate fat burning. Most notable among these are **GLA** (gamma linoleic acid) and **EPA** (eicosapentanoic acid). It now appears that the reason drinking safflower oil made Dr. Taller lose weight is because in individuals of normal metabolism, the linoleic acid in the safflower oil is converted to GLA, which stimulates fat burning. One of the *many* biochemical differences between those of normal weight and the chronically obese may be that obese people's bodies do not perform this conversion. In clinical studies, supplements of GLA resulted in fat loss for many subjects. You can buy GLA as capsules of either evening primrose oil or borage oil. I take evening primrose oil capsules daily.

Another oil that has been helpful for fat burning in many people is **flax seed oil,** which contains EPA, just as fish oil does. I've recommended this elsewhere, and repeat here that I think flax seed oil, or, better yet, flax seed meal, is a fine addition to your low-carb diet.

One more oil that has some pretty strong clinical studies backing up its fat-burning abilities is conjugated linoleic acid, also known as **CLA.** or "Tonalin." There are a fair number of studies published in medical journals showing that this oil causes an increase in fat burning, while helping your body to hang on to muscle tissue. Furthermore, CLA appears to help prevent cancer. I take CLA, too. Personally, I haven't noticed any drastic weight loss effect, but I have heard from a few readers who found that this oil made the difference between a perpetual plateau and weight loss.

- Go paleo. Drop not only dairy, but also soy, cashews, coffee, alcohol, vinegar, artificial sweeteners—everything in your diet that wouldn't have been available to a caveman. As a consolation, you get a bit more fruit. This has worked very well for several people I've been in touch with. Once again, if you're looking for a guide, I recommend Ray Audette's *Neanderthin*.

- Up your exercise, or change it. If you're currently not getting any exercise at all, adding just a fifteen-minute walk each day could make a big difference. If you're already exercising regularly, keep in mind this piece of info from my trainer friend BJ: After about six to eight weeks, your body is accustomed to whatever workout you've been doing, and your returns will diminish. If you've been using a treadmill, try doing aerobics; if you've been doing aerobics, try circuit training instead. Mix it up. And remember: Aerobic exercise burns calories while you're doing it. Resistance training, by increasing your muscle mass, helps you burn more calories twenty-four hours a day.
- Related to exercising, breathe. I've been doing breathing exercises for a couple of years, and they've done good things for my body. Fat only burns in the presence of oxygen. If you're exercising, deliberately "force" your breathing—breathe deeper and harder than you think you need to—in through the nose, out through the mouth, and concentrate on emptying your lungs completely, to make room for fresh air.
- Get your thyroid checked. If you have a slow thyroid, all efforts to lose weight will be in vain. You may also well be tired, chilly, depressed, have a low sex drive, brittle hair, constipation, headaches, cloudy thinking, and you'll heal slowly and have a poor immune system. Not fun.
  There's a safe, easy, free way to find out if you're hypothyroid (have low thyroid function): Take your temperature in your armpit first thing in the morning, before you get out of bed. It's best not to do this during the first couple of days of a menstrual period, which affects temperature. Tuck a thermometer in your armpit, and leave it there for ten minutes. If it reads less than 97.8, you just might be hypothyroid. If it reads under 96.8, you very likely are. (This is called the Broda Barnes Basal Metabolism Test, by the way.)

- Go see a doctor you trust, and *insist* that he or she take this seriously. Be aware that there is such a thing as "sub-clinical" hypothyroidism—a low-level deficiency that does-n't show up on lab tests but will cause a low temperature and keep you from losing weight and feeling well. If you have the symptoms listed above, and your morning temper-ature tests low, find a doctor who will help!
- Cut the caffeine. Caffeine can cause a rise in blood sugar! It triggers the adrenal glands to release hormones that, in turn, release stored sugar into the bloodstream. This is why many low-carb diets ban caffeine.

On the other hand, I have a cup of tea—with caffeine—in front of me as I write this. And many, many folks find that they do just fine on a low-carb diet without ever giving up caffeine. Further, caffeine is recommended by some as a "thermogenic" to stimulate fat burning! Confusing, huh?

I wouldn't be in a huge hurry to drop caffeine, but if you find that you're hungry within an hour of drinking a caffeinat-ed beverage, you may be sensitive. The solution, of course, is to give it up. Easier said than done! Caffeine withdrawal can be a real bear, causing killer headaches. If you feel that caffeine is limiting your weight loss, I would suggest that you start mixing regular and decaf coffee, or regular and decaf tea, and over the space of a few weeks slowly decrease the level of caffeine, taper-ing off gradually. If you're a cola drinker, you could alternate caffeinated diet cola and decaf, until you're drinking all decaf.

I drink half-caf tea myself, except for first thing in the morn-ing. Now that I don't eat carbs, my energy level is so high I can't tolerate fully caffeinated tea all day like I used to.

- Adjust your carb intake—either down or up. I've talked with folks who had to drop their carbs all the way down to 15 grams a day to lose, and I've also heard from folks who had better results when they bumped their carbs up to 60 or 70 grams.
- Count calories. Yes, I know it doesn't seem fair that you should have to pay attention to carbs and calories both, but I've heard from quite a few people for whom this was

necessary. If you do decide to count calories, don't decide to cut back drastically. This can easily backfire on you. Your metabolism may well drop, which isn't the effect we're looking for! You may also end up hungry and miserable, which is a good way to quit your diet altogether. How many calories do you need? Rule of thumb: twelve to fifteen calories per day for every pound of what would be your healthy weight. Note: "Healthy weight" does not mean the weight that you wish that Nature had granted you, the weight that would make you a size 2. It means just that—a reasonable, healthy weight for your body, even if that weight wouldn't make you look fashionably anorexic.

- Pay attention to possible food sensitivities. A year after I went low carb, my husband and I went on a camping trip. Thinking I could avoid preparing lunches, I bought a big bag of peanuts in the shell, reasoning that the shells would force me to eat them more slowly than shelled peanuts, and that with the exercise I would get while camping (we walk several miles a day while camping, as a rule), the carbohydrates in the peanuts wouldn't be a big problem.

Imagine my chagrin when I got home after a three-day trip—and had gained seven or eight pounds!

I continued to eat peanuts, although I was careful about quantities. It wasn't until a couple of years later that I realized that quantity wasn't the problem!

One night while watching TV, a few hours after dinner, my husband brought out a can of peanuts. I had two small handfuls —and within minutes I was wheezing slightly. I could feel my waistband cutting into me uncomfortably, and suddenly my wedding ring was tight. I was allergic to peanuts!

I cut the peanuts out of my diet entirely—a sad thing to do; I love them. But I found that I had far fewer sudden swings in weight after I eliminated them from my diet. I haven't managed to maintain that complete ban on peanuts, especially when developing recipes! But still, when I avoid them, I have a much easier time keeping my weight under control.

Hidden food sensitivities can torpedo your weight loss. They can also be the source of fierce food cravings. There is a phenomenon called "allergic-addiction." This means that the foods you are most likely to be allergic to are the ones you crave most and eat most often! (I was eating a nut-and-seed mix with peanuts in it almost every day.) The uncomfortable symptoms of the allergy—headaches, fatigue, spaciness, depression, etc.—start to set in as you withdraw from the food, and you crave the food to stop the symptoms. But it can only make you worse in the long run, just like sugar.

The most commonly allergic/addictive foods are the grains (corn, wheat, rye, oats, rice), soy, milk and dairy products, yeast, eggs, citrus fruits, shellfish, nuts, and chocolate. However, you can be sensitive to anything!

If you're quite sure you've got your carb intake under control but you still have unpleasant symptoms an hour or so after eating and can't lose weight, you may have a food sensitivity.

How to find out? The simplest way is to drop the suspected food—and remember, it's likely to be one of the foods you eat and crave the most—from your diet for three or four weeks and see how you feel. Then, if you like, you can add it back and see if the symptoms reappear. You may be surprised! It's not uncommon for people to feel heavily drugged when they eat an allergenic food after not having it for a while.

Another way to find out is to eat the suspected food, all by itself, on an empty stomach. Wait several hours from your last meal. Then, before you eat the suspected food, take your pulse. (Find it at your neck or wrist, count it for fifteen seconds by the clock, and then multiply by four.) Eat a moderate-sized portion of the food you're testing. Remain seated, and take your pulse again at five, ten, and fifteen minutes. What you're looking for is a speeding up of your pulse. If you get one, that's a clue that particular food may not be great for your body.

An alternative indicator can be a change in handwriting after eating a suspected food. Once again, you test after fasting for several hours. Write your name as clearly as you can, eat the suspected food, wait ten or fifteen minutes, and write your name again. If there is deterioration in your handwriting, I'd drop that food, fast!

You can, of course, talk to a doctor about this. If you do so, be aware that most doctors only accept a certain kind of sensitivity—to be technical, one that is "IgE antibody mediated"—as a true allergy. Most food sensitivities don't fall into this category. Tests for "IgG antibody" response, or "cytotoxic" testing, are likely to be closer to the mark. You may have to search to find a doctor who will do these tests. Don't let yourself be intimidated! Remember, doctors work for *you*!

But I'd start by paying attention to which foods you crave most, and noticing how your body reacts when you eat that food alone, on an empty stomach.

- Take a look at your medications. It is very, very common for women to gain weight when they start taking birth control pills or estrogen replacement therapy (ERT). I've seen friends balloon by twenty-five pounds in a matter of months!

This is because estrogen encourages fat deposition and water retention. That's why women have a much harder time losing weight than men do! It's also why farmers give beef cattle artificial estrogens; it makes them gain weight.

What can you do? First of all, if you can possibly tolerate a birth control method other than those that affect hormones—the Pill, the birth control patch, or Depo-Provera—your body will thank you for it by losing weight. These all are unbalancing and have weight gain as a side effect.

If it is *essential* that you use hormonally based birth control—for instance, pregnancy would be disastrous, but you're deeply morally opposed to abortion—you might consider supplementing progesterone as well. You can consult your doctor, if you like. Some women find this helps with the estrogen weight gain.

Another possibility for those who take hormone replacement therapy (HRT) is to consider taking pregnenolone instead. As mentioned before, this is a hormone "precursor"; a substance your body uses to make many different hormones from. When you take this precursor, your body decides just how much estrogen it wants to make, how much progesterone, how much testosterone (yes, women have testosterone, too; it's responsible for our sex drive), how much of the other hormones. This strikes me as a far more balanced, natural approach to hormone supplementation. Since your body makes DHEA from pregnenolone, you could, if you like, get a DHEA saliva test from your doctor to see if you really need it, or you can simply try a small dose—maybe 10 to 30 milligrams—in place of your HRT for a few months to see what the results are. DON'T TAKE THE PREGNENOLONE—OR DHEA—ALONG WITH HRT! Overkill! And *do* let your doctor know what you're doing and why.

- Stop drinking. As I have mentioned, I have a couple of glasses of dry wine or a couple of light beers every evening. However, I don't consider this optimal for weight loss, whether on a low-carb diet or any other diet.

Despite the fact that my wine and beer have only 3 to 4 grams of carbohydrate per serving, and distilled liquor has none (one popular low-carb diet of the 1960s was called *The Drinking Man's Diet* because it allowed distilled liquor, on the theory it had no carbs), they're still a *major* luxury. Why? Because chemically speaking, alcohol is closer to carbohydrate than it is to anything else. There's little question that alcohol slows metabolism, making it harder to lose weight. I'm quite certain if I gave it up I'd drop several more pounds.

But I *like* my wine and beer! And especially where the wine is concerned, there's a lot of evidence that it has other beneficial effects on health—even some evidence that dry red wines improve insulin utilization!

This is another one where you'll have to see how your body reacts. If you like alcohol, and you can have a little (notice the word *little!*) and still lose weight, great! If you include alcohol and you're not losing, it's one of the most likely culprits.

Watch out which wines and beers you choose! Dry wines include Chablis, Rhine, pinot noir, gewürztraminer, sauvignon blanc, cabernet sauvignon, burgundy, merlot, Chianti. If you're not *certain* that a wine is dry, ask the liquor store clerk or the waiter. Sweet wines can have a *lot* of sugar in them! And even the dry wines can vary in carbohydrate content quite a lot from brand to brand. If you can't find the brand you want in your food count book, consider calling the company. I did this with Franzia vineyards, and they were very helpful. Just explain that you have a medical condition that requires that you avoid carbs.

Light beers vary *tremendously* in carbohydrate count. Most of them are so high in carbs I won't drink them—7 grams a can or so—which, high as it is, is still only *half* of what most regular beers have! But there are a few light beers that run between 3 and 4 grams per can. *Those* are the ones you want. Do I have to say it again? READ THE LABEL! (If you're ordering a light beer while out, remember that Miller Light has far fewer carbs than Bud Light.)

Most plain distilled liquors have no actual carbs in them—whisky, scotch, vodka, gin, tequila, and rum fall into this category. Beyond these, however, danger looms! Just about all liqueurs, cordials, flavored schnapps, etc., have a *ton* of sugar in them. So do most mixers—whiskey sour mix, margarita mix, daiquiri mix, piña colada mix, orange juice, you name it. And wine coolers are right out! If you want a mixed drink, try a gin and tonic made with *diet* tonic water (yes, tonic has sugar!), or a rum and cola made with diet cola. A Bloody Mary now and then is *just* passable; tomato juice is lower in carbs than fruit juices.

Club soda and sparkling water are carb free, of course, so you could have a scotch and soda. Or you could have my favorite "tall" drink, a wine spritzer. I put about three ounces of burgundy in a tall glass with ice and fill it up with berry-flavored sparkling water. This actually tastes sweet to me, despite the very low carb count.

Still, alcohol on any diet has to be considered a luxury. Be aware of this, and choose accordingly.

And last but not least:

- Ask yourself if you really need to lose more weight. Are

you healthy? Energetic? Blood work looks good? Immune
system strong? Knees and back don't ache? Reasonable,
attractive size? If you're a size 10 or 8, and you're trying to
get down to a 4, your body may be telling you that you're
not supposed to be that small. My body seems to think I
should be a size 12. I may eventually get down as small as
a 10, but I doubt I'll ever be an 8, much less a 4. It is my
observation that a low-carbohydrate diet is very useful for
fixing genuine obesity and avoiding the dreadful medical
problems that come with it, but is not well suited for
becoming unhealthily thin. If your aim is to become fashionably anorexic looking, I can't help you.

CHAPTER TWENTY-TWO

Enhancing Success

For Emotional Eaters—Saint John's Wort, 5-hydroxytryptophan, Niacin

Is there anybody left who doesn't know that Saint John's Wort is a natural, herbal antidepressant? Prescribed twice as often as pharmaceutical antidepressants in Europe, and proven effective in clinical tests. Fairly cheap, too!

Why mention this antidepressant in a diet book? Because there's a pretty fair argument to be made that one of the things that makes people crave carbohydrates is the fact that taking on a big load of starch and/or sugar will rapidly raise brain levels of a chemical called serotonin. And serotonin is a mood elevator— the way Prozac and similar drugs work is by raising brain levels of serotonin.

Unfortunately, the effect on serotonin from eating carbs is short-lived, just like the blood sugar rush, and you're left tired and irritable and craving more. Not good!

So, raising your brain levels of serotonin in *other* ways can be a good strategy for you if you're prone to or depression- or stress-related binging. All three of the substances in the heading above—Saint John's Wort, 5-hydroxytryptophan, and niacin— can do that for you.

They work in different ways, and I know people—myself occasionally included—who take all three.

Saint John's Wort, it's beginning to appear, works in a similar fashion to Prozac. Prozac falls into a class of drugs called SSRIs, which stands for "Selective Serotonin Reuptake Inhibitors." Let me explain.

Each of your brain cells has a microscopic space, called a *synapse,* between it and the next cell. Messages are sent from one cell to the next by chemicals, called *neurotransmitters,* that flow in and fill the space, and then are immediately pumped back out again so they can be reused. Serotonin is one of those neurotransmitters. Prozac and other SSRIs slow down the pumping out/recycling mechanism, so that serotonin, which makes us feel cheerful and calm, stimulates the brain cells longer. It's beginning to appear that Saint John's Wort works in much the same way.

Be aware that high doses of Saint John's Wort may cause photosensitivity—in other words, you'll sunburn more easily. If you decide to try it, keep this in mind and don't forget to protect yourself.

Then there's 5-hydroxytryptophan. This is what your body uses to make serotonin out of, so taking it, especially on an empty stomach, can increase brain levels of serotonin. Good to take before bed; it can help you get a good night's sleep, with no hangover.

You may well have heard of tryptophan. It's an amino acid found in many protein foods. A lot of people blame post-Thanksgiving dinner sleepiness on tryptophan. And supplements of tryptophan were popular as an insomnia and depression treatment in the 1980s, until a contaminated batch lead to illness and a number of deaths, and tryptophan supplements were banned. Also called 5-HTP, 5-hydroxytryptophan works similarly.

The way I understand it, your body turns tryptophan into 5-hydroxytryptophan, and *then* into serotonin—the 5-HTP is the intermediate step. So the difference in effect on serotonin levels is minimal. When I looked through the medical journal database, I found studies that showed that 5-HTP worked as well as Prozac and Paxil for treating mild to moderate depression and anxiety.

Then there's niacin. Niacin is a B vitamin, B3 to be exact. Niacin has some profound effects on brain chemistry, to say the least! For instance, Dr. Abram Hoffer worked with schizophrenics, and found that for many of them, huge doses of niacin would lessen or eliminate the psychosis. He theorized that many schizophrenics simply had an abnormally high need for niacin.

For that matter, it was common folk wisdom in the 1960s and 1970s that if someone was having a bad acid trip, you could pull them right out of it by giving them a big dose of niacin. Set their scrambled brain chemicals right, fast!

Niacin also can lessen cravings for nicotine. The proper, scientific name for niacin is "nicotinic acid," and its calming effect on the brain is not unlike that of tobacco.

All of these effects seem to relate to niacin's ability to increase brain levels of serotonin. You see, when you eat tryptophan in food (remember, it's an amino acid and it's present in many protein foods we eat), your body can use that tryptophan to make *either* niacin or serotonin. If you're short on niacin—and evidence is that different people can need different amounts—your body uses the tryptophan for niacin, not serotonin. If you take plenty of niacin, your body is more likely to use the tryptophan for serotonin.

One warning about niacin: Vitamin B3 comes in two forms, niacin and niacinamide. They both have about the same effect on your moods. The difference between the two is that niacin causes a "flush"—about fifteen to twenty minutes after you take niacin, all your surface blood vessels dilate, and you become hot, red, and itchy all over! This flush lasts for about fifteen minutes and is harmless. Personally, I kinda like it! But some people find it very irritating or even frightening. When I worked in the health food store, I used to have people return niacin, explaining that they were terribly allergic to it!

The niacin flush does have some benefits. The same chemical that causes the flush also causes allergic reactions: histamine. (When you have allergies, you take antihistamines, right? That's because allergic symptoms—runny nose, itchy eyes, hives, sneezing—are caused by histamine.) The niacin flush is like a temporary case of the hives. By deliberately dumping histamine stores on a daily basis, some people find that their allergies become milder.

Also, only niacin, with its flush, will *lower cholesterol*. Niacin is a fairly potent cholesterol-lowering substance, proven in many clinical trials. However, it seems to have an effect on cholesterol only in *very* big doses, between a gram and 3 grams a day—for comparison, I take 100 milligrams, or a tenth of a gram, daily. If you're blue *and* have high cholesterol, you may want to try niacin in larger doses. But DON'T DO IT WITHOUT YOUR DOCTOR'S SUPERVISION. At doses of 1 to 3 grams a day, niacin is more a drug than a vitamin, and has been known to cause liver inflammation in susceptible people.

For purposes of raising your serotonin levels, I'd stay with 100–250 milligrams, once or twice a day. And for this purpose, you can take niacinamide instead and avoid the flush entirely.

All three of these substances—Saint John's Wort, 5-HTP, and niacin—are pretty darn safe. But don't be a dope! It's your brain you're playing around with here, *for heavens sake!* So take care. If you're under treatment for profound depression, please *don't* try to go off of your antidepressant drugs and switch over to any of these three without a doctor's input!

Also know that for every substance in the world there's *someone* who reacts badly to it. I used to baby-sit a little boy who was allergic to breastmilk! The point is, if you start taking one or more of these substances and feel *worse* instead of better, pay attention!

None of these three serotonin-raising, mood-elevating substances will actually speed up your weight loss. But they can make it far easier to go low carb and stick to it! If you find yourself reaching for candy or bread or ice cream when you're feeling blue, these three substances may be for you.

Thermogenics

Remember what I said about naturally skinny people having bodies that simply turn up the heat and burn off excess calories? Guess what! There are over-the-counter drugs and herbal preparations that will up your body temperature slightly and help burn off fat. We call these products "thermogenics." And my experience is that they do work—but that there are some real dangers involved, so caution is *essential*.

The most commonly used thermogenic agent is called *ephedrine*. Ephedrine has been widely used for decades for asthma; it's a major ingredient in Primatene tablets. It's also a decongestant. Ephedrine is also popular as an over-the-counter pep pill. I often see ephedrine at truck stops, since truckers use it to stay awake on long runs. Interestingly, the brand I see most often at truck stops is called "Mini Thin," a reference to the thermogenic effect. Ephedrine also is sometimes sold by the tablet on the black market as cheap speed, called "white cross," a reference to the double-scoring, or cross mark, on the tablets.

Ephedrine is currently pretty controversial stuff, largely because a few morons have gotten stupid with it. Kids looking for kicks will take outrageous doses, and illegal drug labs will combine it with other chemicals, including *Drano* for heaven's sake, to produce much more powerful and dangerous forms of speed, including methcathinone and methamphetamine. (On its own, ephedrine is *much* milder than either of these illegal drugs.) There has been some talk of removing ephedrine from the market, or making it available only by prescription. I have noticed that it now seems to be combined with guafenisin, a drug that loosens up phlegm, whenever I see it. Apparently this prevents people from misusing it somehow.

How does ephedrine work? It's a *sympathomimetic,* meaning it mimics the effects of adrenaline in the body. It increases heart rate, opens up the breathing passages (which is why it's effective for asthma and colds), and makes you feel energetic or jittery, depending on how much you take. It also increases the metabolic rate of fat tissue, which is what we like about it! Some adrenal hormones encourage fat burning; there's speculation that one of the differences between people who are naturally slim and those of us who gain easily may be in levels of adrenal hormones. Again, ephedrine increases your body temperature very slightly (not enough to notice; you won't be sweating all the time or anything), so you burn off more calories, even when you're sitting still.

Side effects include increased blood pressure, insomnia, anxiety, and reduced appetite. In most people who use moderate doses, the insomnia, anxiety, and appetite suppression wear off in a week or so. However, the thermogenic (fat burning) effect remains. Some even feel the fat-burning effect increases with time!

Ephedrine works best in combination with two other drugs you're familiar with: caffeine and aspirin. I don't understand the chemistry, but all the clinical studies show that these two drugs increase the fat-burning effectiveness of ephedrine quite a bit. This combination of drugs is usually referred to as a "stack," or "ECA stack." The most commonly recommended dose is 20–25 milligrams of ephedrine (most tablets are this strength), a cup of coffee or one No-Doz or Vivarin tablet, and half an aspirin (some feel a baby aspirin—a quarter of an aspirin—is enough), three times a day.

Personally, that's way too much ephedrine for me! I've taken the stuff, and I've found that a full 25-milligram ephedrine tablet is enough to make me want to jump right out of my skin. Furthermore, taking it in the morning and afternoon is okay, but if I take an evening dose, no *way* am I going to sleep! When I've used pharmaceutical ephedrine, I've taken half to three-quarters of a tablet (about 12 to 19 milligrams), with a pot of tea and half an aspirin. Tea, by the way, has a thermogenic effect of its own, as we'll discuss in a minute.

If you want to buy plain old pharmaceutical ephedrine, in double-scored white cross tablets, you may be able to find it at a truck stop or gas station. You sometimes find ads for mail-order ephedrine in exercise magazines. If you want to increase effectiveness by "stacking," add to that a bottle of baby aspirin and some source of caffeine, whether a beverage or No-Doz or Vivarin tablets. This would be your least expensive option.

There's an easier way to do this, although it's not quite as inexpensive. *Many* companies now put out herbal versions of the ECA stack, with all three substances in one tablet, often with other ingredients included. The herbal version of ephedrine— which, of course, was the original, and which has been used in herbal medicine for centuries —is called *ma huang* (pronounced mah wong) or *ephedra*. It is the main ingredient in many herbal pep pills and most herbal diet pills. In most herbal thermogenics, guarana is used to supply caffeine, and willow bark is used to supply an aspirinlike compound. These products work about the same as the ephedrine/caffeine/aspirin combo, but many people are more comfortable with the idea of taking herbs.

There are also herbal ephedrine products that include some herbal diuretics, like uva ursi. Since a low-carb diet will itself reduce water retention, I think these are not for us. Some products also include herbal laxatives like cascara sagrada, which I consider a very bad idea. And I've seen one or two products that combine ma huang with Saint John's Wort to speed fat burning *and* cut emotional carb cravings. This may be useful.

There is some feeling that prolonged use of ephedrine can be hard on the adrenal glands; some of the herbal products include herbs like licorice that supposedly prevent this effect. I'm not knowledgeable enough to be able to say whether this is effective or not. Also, there is some feeling that it is best to cycle on and off thermogenics, taking them for a week, then taking a day or two off, and then starting again. This is said to prevent some of the weakening of the adrenal glands, and to prevent your body's adapting to the ephedrine and its losing effectiveness.

I feel that ephedrine and ma huang can be useful adjuncts to your low-carb diet, to maximize fat burning and increase energy. However, these are *powerful drugs*—yes, even the herbs are *drugs*—and must be used with sense and caution! If you use them recklessly, they can make you very uncomfortable, or *even kill you. So don't be stupid.*

First of all, if you have high blood pressure, heart disease, clots, *any* cardiovascular condition at all, ephedrine/ma huang is NOT FOR YOU. It could give you a heart attack or a stroke. If

you are taking MAO inhibitors, or any other prescription medication, for that matter, I'd avoid it. If you're prone to seizures,
it's a bad idea as well. I knew a young man who was seizure-
prone who gave himself a seizure by taking large doses of
ephedrine. If you have glaucoma, ephedrine is a no-no. And, like
any drug, ephedrine should not be taken during pregnancy or if
you are breast-feeding. (Tangentially, breast-feeding will dramatically speed weight loss after pregnancy, especially in your
butt and thighs. It's not just much better for your baby, it's much
better for you, too.) Furthermore, you shouldn't take ephedrine
or ma huang if you have thyroid disease or if you're a man with
prostate trouble.

**Do NOT decide that if a little ephedrine is good, a lot will
be better.** Again, it is not unknown for people—even healthy
young people—to *die* of overdoses of the stuff, just like any other
drug, and the fact that it's available without a prescription or as a
"natural, herbal" product does *not* change that. I would *strongly*
caution you not to take any product that gives you more than 25
milligrams of ephedrine in a dose, and I personally would not
take more than three doses in a day. (That being said, at this
writing I have on hand a popular herbal thermogenic from a
network marketing company. It contains 22 milligrams of
"ephedrine activity" per capsule, and the instructions suggest
taking two at a time. I won't do it, no matter what their label
says. I'm sure I'd drop weight if I did, but I consider it risky, and
anyway, I'd never be able to sit still and write this book!)

Having now effectively scared you to death, let me say that
ephedrine and ma huang are substances that have been used
safely for centuries. Ephedrine has been classified as a non-
prescription drug for decades, and authorities have only been
deeply concerned about it in the past ten years or so, when
people have started abusing it. Used with caution and good
sense, I feel that for healthy people, ephedrine can be a safe and
effective diet aid.

There is an alternative to ephedrine/ma huang, however.
Recently, bitter orange has been found to have chemicals that
have a similar effect to ephedrine/ma huang—they cause

thermogenesis and fat burning. Since the FDA has become alarmed about ephedrine abuse, some herbal and nutritional supplement companies have been switching over to the bitter orange thermogenics. Bitter orange extracts are felt to be less stimulating or "speedy," but to still be effective for fat burning. I plan to try a bitter orange–based thermogenic soon. The same precautions that apply to ephedrine products also apply to bitter orange products.

Tea, Green and Otherwise

Surely you've heard by now that green tea is good for you—it's loaded with antioxidants that slow the aging process and reduce your risk of cancer and heart disease. Well, here are two more pieces of good news: Tea also increases fat burning—and it's not just green tea that's good for you!

Green tea and black tea (what we think of as "regular" tea) come from the same plant, it's just that for black tea the leaves are fermented, and for green tea they're not. There's a third kind you may not have heard of, called oolong tea, which is partially fermented—somewhere between green tea and black tea. All three kinds of tea—green, black, and oolong—are the healthiest beverages you can imagine. The antioxidants in tea help prevent cancer and heart disease, slow the aging process, and even lower cholesterol levels. (This gives me great joy. I am a lifelong tea addict, and back when I worked in a holistic health center, my veggie-organic colleagues would say, "You shouldn't drink tea! It has caffeine! It has tannic acid! You should drink *herb* tea!" And I would say, "NO! Tea is my friend! Tea wouldn't hurt me! My Aunt Grace wouldn't have given me tea if it were bad for me!" When the news came out about tea's dramatic health-giving properties, I was pretty darned smug, I can tell you.)

Well, it turns out that antioxidants are only the half of it. I have in front of me a medical journal article regarding "green tea extract," showing that people treated with the extract burned 4 percent more calories over twenty-four hours than people who simply were given caffeine or a placebo. Another study showed that green tea stimulated metabolism far more than could be explained by its caffeine content. In other words, the tea itself is a thermogenic!

Another study showed more than a 4 percent decrease in body weight, and a reduction of 4.5 percent in waist size in three months, simply because of green tea extract.

But as I said, it's not just the green tea. In another study, oolong tea "demonstrated...anti-obesity effects." It appears that tea, in general, is a useful tool in our struggle to stay slim and fit.

You can, of course, drink tea, and I would urge you to do so—especially if tea is replacing diet soda and other artificially flavored and sweetened beverages in your diet. Hot or iced, brewed or from instant tea powder, tea is a far healthier beverage than anything that comes in a can or a bottle. (You can, of course, buy artificially flavored and sweetened iced tea in bottles, and it should have some of the beneficial chemicals in it, but then you're back to the artificial sweeteners and citric acid that block weight loss in some low-carb dieters.) I've also read reports of folks who switched from coffee to tea for their caffeine fix and spontaneously lost a few pounds. If you don't like caffeine, remember that it's not just the caffeine in tea that helps you lose weigh—you can drink decaf and get much of the beneficial effect.

If you simply can't abide tea, there are capsules of green tea extract available—look at your local health food store. These capsules should be effective, and safer than ephedrine.

Time to go brew another pot!

Other Helpful Stuff

L-Glutamine

L-glutamine is an amino acid—one of those protein "letters" we talked about. Supplements of pure l-glutamine help many people overcome carb cravings during the first few weeks of low carbing, by making it easier for your body to create what little sugar it does need. Since you get a steadier level of glucose in your bloodstream, you get far fewer carb cravings.

L-glutamine has also been shown to raise levels of growth

hormone in the bloodstream, which can help you burn fat and build muscle. To get this effect, you need to take at least two grams of l-glutamine on an empty stomach either right before working out or right before going to sleep.

A third benefit of l-glutamine that has nothing to do with weight loss is that it often improves memory, especially in the middle-aged to elderly.

You can buy l-glutamine capsules at a health food store. There are also beverages that are made especially for low carbers that include l-glutamine to fight carb cravings. The "Keto" line of products has a few of these. If you have nasty carb cravings, either capsules or one of these beverages are worth seeking out.

L-Carnitine

L-carnitine is controversial—some people, including Dr. Atkins, say it assists fat burning by helping fat get into the cell to be burned for energy. Others, including many of the medical journal articles I was able to find on the subject, say it doesn't help weight loss at all. For that matter, l-carnitine is one of the main ingredients in Pentabosol, the weight loss supplement marketed by Drs. Michael and Mary Dan Eades. I tried Pentabosol and got no results to speak of. When I looked at the Fitness Infomercial Review Web site (www.fitnessinfomercialreview.com), most people said that they, too, had little to no result with Pentabosol— but one woman said she'd lost twelve pounds since she started taking it. And Dr. Atkins said that high doses of l-carnitine—a few grams a day—help to overcome metabolic resistance to weight loss.

Seems to be a real "your mileage may vary" issue, but if you're having trouble losing weight on your low-carb diet, l-carnitine is worth a try. Find it at your health food store, or order Pentabosol from the infomercial or the Eadeses' Web site.

CHAPTER TWENTY-THREE

Exercise

WHAT WOULD A weight-loss book be without the obligatory chapter on exercise? You know it's good for you, you know you should—but statistics say you probably don't do it. This is my attempt to change that!

Exercise will give you energy, raise your spirits, create glucagon to help you release fat for burning, speed your metabolism, and all around improve your life. It will make you feel better about yourself, your body, and the world. It will, to a large degree, slow and even reverse the aging process, since much of what we think of as the ravages of aging are really the results of gradual muscle loss. If God hadn't invented exercise, some big corporation would be charging you $60 a shot to take a walk! Or as one wag put it, "We've found the magic anti-aging pill. It just takes 20 minutes three times a week to swallow it."

But forget that stuff. Here's the bottom line: Exercise will improve the way you *look* about a thousand percent. For most of us, that's our *real* motivation for doing any of this. When I've lectured on low-carb dieting, it's been very clear that the people who came to hear me were concerned about appearance first, with health a distant second.

We want to be attractive. We want to be appealing. We want to be noticed. We want to be *sexy*.

Maybe people shouldn't judge each other by the way we look. But we do. We do. And we all live with it. Women in particular—we're constantly comparing ourselves to surgically augmented, airbrushed super models (most of whom work out, by the way!), and we have the nasty suspicion that the rest of the world is, too—and all too often, they are. We women obsess about our weight because on some level it stands for our whole sense of self-worth as a woman. Men do diet, do worry about their weight and their looks, but it's not with the same desperate feeling women have.

(For the men reading this: If you'd like to understand why we women are so psycho about our weight, try to imagine growing up in a world where every magazine, every TV station, all your life, told you over and over that if you just had "willpower" and "strength of character" and "self-esteem" enough to torture and starve yourself the rest of your life, you could make your penis bigger. Now imagine this in a society where your penis was on display every time you went out of the house. Get it?)

Exercise *shows*. Everything pulls up and in. You move better. Your skin looks healthier. You stand with more confidence. You move with purpose. You feel sexy. You *look* sexy! (Not while you're doing it; in between times!) *Everyone* notices on some level.

Your posture improves. Standing straight and tall, torso lifted up out of your hips, shoulders square, stomach taut, neck long—gets rid of ten pounds and ten years, at least! But you can't achieve this, and feel comfortable with it, without *exercise*. Your muscles simply won't be up to the task.

You probably know all of this. Yet the chances are good that you're *still* not exercising! Especially if, like me, you've had weight and energy problems all your life, gym class was probably the most humiliating part of your childhood. So here's a little inspiration for you to get out and get moving!

Pep Talk for Gym-Class Dropouts

I am one of you. When I was fifteen and a high school sopho-more, I cut an entire semester of gym. Didn't even go to day one. Got a "C," too, though only God (and the bureaucracy) knows how! (Ridgewood High, please don't call!) I was a reader and a talker, not an athlete of any kind.

Sports, games, exercise—to me these were NOT fun; they were sheer humiliation. The phrase I heard over and over and over again on the elementary school playground, as sides were chosen for dodgeball or kickball or prison, was, "And you get Carpender!" Not pretty.

(To any elementary school teachers reading this: If you are still using the "choosing up sides" method of establishing teams, I implore you to *cut it out!* I am sure that this torture alone is responsible for thousands of adult sports-phobics. Have 'em count off, one-two, one-two, instead.)

I was, as I have said, fat by the age of eight or nine. I was not—still am not—very coordinated. I was the kid who could never make it up the rope. I was the kid who missed the easy throws and took a softball in the eye. I was the kid who was too fat and slow to get away from the dodgeball. I was the kid who never really understood the rules of any game, and made stupid, embarrassing mistakes as a result.

Yet at the age of forty-five, I am *fit*. I exercise regularly, and I actually *enjoy* it. I am convinced that anyone can do the same. There are just three things you need to understand to make exer-cise a part of your life.

Number one: If you, like me, have associated all things ath-letic with severe humiliation, you need to know a very important fact: No one is going to make fun of you if you're not a great athlete! Maybe you'll want to avoid team sports—I do—but as far as the world of adult exercise goes, the simple fact that you're *trying* is enough to make you one of the gang, one of the elite. Effort counts for *everything*; skill for very little. No one cares how you look in your workout clothes, either. I promise you, I have never been to a gym where people were even the tini-est bit mean about people who weren't as athletic as they. Really.

You don't have to play a game, *ever,* to get in shape. And you never have to compete with anybody but yourself. Furthermore, I've gone to aerobics class as a size 18, in shiny pink spandex, and not a single person made fun of me. Not one! Grownups, thank God, are kinder about these things than kids are.

Number two: Anything that keeps you moving around at a pretty good clip counts as exercise! You don't have to join a gym if you don't want to. You simply need to move around! If you rake your yard for forty-five minutes—assuming you keep moving instead of stopping and starting—*that's* an aerobic exercise. So is walking. So is dancing. If you spend all Saturday lifting rocks and putting them into place for a patio or rock garden, that's both aerobic and strength training! You may not want to get on a stair climber, but how about going out Latin dancing a couple of times a week? The trick is to come up with something that you actually find not hideously unpleasant, and then *do* it. Regularly!

Number three: Exercise will make you *feel great*! And it will make you look better, fast. I'm not making it up. Really. One of the great things about exercise is that it's the only totally reliable thing I know: If you do it, it works. Period. Not, if you do it and the weather holds out, it works, or if you do it and your boss approves, it works, or if you do it and you can get the funding, it works. If you exercise, you *will* get stronger. And stronger *feels* and *looks* better.

Stronger is not panting as you hustle up the stairs. Stronger is being able to carry in the groceries in two trips, not four. Stronger is being able to dance for hours! Strong is sexy! (All the stars you think of as "naturally" gorgeous are working out, never doubt it!) Stronger is breaking into a trot as you cross the street, just because you feel energetic. Strong IS energetic. And lack of energy is the single greatest health complaint Americans have! If you've been avoiding exercise because you don't have the energy, you're taking exactly the *wrong* approach!

And here's the kicker: If you haven't been exercising at all, you will get *far* more good out of starting even a modest exercise program than a professional athlete would get out of adding another several hours a week! That's right. All of the research shows that the jump in health when you go from no exercise to just twenty or thirty minutes, three or four times a week, is the single greatest gain you can get. Adding another few hours will increase the gain, but not by as much. And for a serious athlete to get any real increase in fitness, he or she would have to add many, many hours, and a great deal of intensity. You're going to get the greatest exercise benefit of all!

So all you have to do is decide which form of exercise is for you. It has to be something you'll actually *do*—no use buying some expensive piece of equipment and ending up using it as a clothes rack. (Been there, done that!)

What is the best kind of exercise? I could talk about the advantages of resistance (weight) training versus aerobics versus anything else—and I will, a bit—but here's what for me is the bottom line:

The best exercise is the one you will *do*!

It doesn't matter if stair-climbing machines burn more calories than walking; if you find walking fun and stair-climbers about as enjoyable as root canal, you'd better go for a walk. I, for one, would rather give a speech to a thousand people dressed only in my old underwear than use a stationary bicycle. This just means that stationary bikes are not for me!

There are three basic classes of exercise: Aerobics, resistance or muscle training, and stretching. These categories can overlap; for instance, many aerobics classes now incorporate work with resistance bands or weights to strengthen muscles. Some stretching programs also strengthen, and things like yoga and Pilates are designed to do both. Weightlifting can be done as "circuit training," where you move from exercise to exercise fast enough that your heart rate doesn't drop, creating aerobic benefits— there's a chain of women's gyms called Curves that works on exactly this principle

Which sort of exercise is most important? Oh, dear. Such a hard call, but I'd like to put in a strong pitch for strength training. During the 1970s and 1980s, aerobics were king. Everyone considered them the most important form of exercise, especially for people who wanted to lose weight. Then new research came in about resistance exercise ("resistance" and "strength" exercise are the same thing—overloading your muscles so that they make themselves stronger as a result), and the picture started to change. We discovered that while aerobics increased your metabolism while you were doing them, and for a little while after, weight training would increase your metabolism *twenty-four hours a day,* even while you're sleeping, by increasing your muscle mass.

Bottom line is that aerobics alone will never reshape your body. Just won't happen. Resistance exercise—weights or resistance bands or resistance training machines—will. If you want the most results in the least amount of time, plus the greatest increase in your metabolism, you'll get that from resistance training. Furthermore, you'll never have to increase the amount of time you work out to increase your results—you just increase the weight or use a heavier band. I love this about resistance! If I wanted to increase my results with a walking program, I'd have to walk more miles, which would take more time. But when I Heavyhand—walk *while doing weight work*—all I have to do to increase my results is add another pound of weight.

Further, a clinical study was done with the elderly. A group of subjects, with an average age well over eighty, was put on a program of progressive resistance exercise. The results? Every single one of them showed an improvement in their ability to stand, walk, balance, climb stairs, and get into and out of chairs. Some who had used walkers for years were able to abandon them! Pretty impressive stuff.

No, ladies, you won't end up looking like a man, or even like a female bodybuilder. Women who look that way work *incredibly* hard, and usually take steroids to get there. You'll just get shapelier. Promise.

I don't want to hear that you have no place or time to exercise. You know and I know you're making excuses. We all do what we really want to do—what we decide is important to us. We find a way, if we really want the benefit. Back when I was working out at a gym, there was a fellow who often was there when I was, mid-40s I'd guess, who had a withered leg, a heavy limp, one hand that curled in and was clearly not fully functional, along with a withered forearm on that side. I had no idea whether this was from an accident or disease or birth defect—but I do know that he was at the gym regularly and in terrific shape. Every muscle not affected by his disability was toned and defined. Then there's my friend Cori, who, after a catastrophic car accident at age seventeen, spent years *crawling* around the track at the local YMCA, getting her strength back so she could learn to walk again. Cori now swims several times a week. For that matter, I've had the good fortune to hear Art Berg, perhaps America's finest motivational speaker. Art is a quadriplegic—and did a 325-mile super-marathon in his wheelchair! We find a way to do what is important to us. NO EXCUSES!

Gym Versus Home

Should you go to the gym, or should you work out at home? Again, a tough call. I've done both, and there are pluses and minuses to each.

Gyms—The Upside

Obviously, a good gym is going to have equipment you don't have at home, including any and all weight training stuff you might need. Gyms can offer a lot of camaraderie, and most of them now have childcare. If you've tried to work out at home but the kids keep interrupting, joining a gym may be the solution. Please don't think you have to wear fancy, sexy workout clothes to go to a gym. I've often worked out at a gym in ancient elastic-waist shorts and old, beat-up T-shirts. There are some "meat market" gyms where everybody dresses up, but in my experience they're few and far between. Just wear something comfortable and good gym shoes.

Many people join gyms to attend classes of various kinds. Almost all gyms will have classes ranging from beginner to advanced, and they'll include aerobic activities like kickboxing and step aerobics—many of which now include some strength work with weights or resistance bands, too (highly recommended)—as well as toning activities like yoga and Pilates. I'd recommend taking classes that both strengthen and increase cardio fitness.

If you decide to take aerobics, please be aware that *everybody* takes a while to catch on to the commands in aerobics class. Everybody looks dopey the first few times they do it. There's no shame in missing your footing or in taking a few weeks to figure it all out. Just keep moving—as my trainer friend BJ would say, "Your heart doesn't know if your feet are doing it right." I did step aerobics for a long time, and I *never* got to the point where I performed every move right. Big deal. Just keep moving!

Another big plus for gyms: You'll find knowledgeable people who can show you the ropes. If you're intimidated by the specialized equipment—many people are—this is a big help! Once you've gone through your routine a few times, it's not complicated at all. If you have concerns about physical limitations, it's also very helpful to talk to people who are certified in athletic training; they can help you put together a program that is safe and effective for you.

If you get bored with the same routine fairly quickly, a gym lets you change your type of workout a lot, without spending extra money for new equipment. You can take aerobics for six weeks, then switch over to the stair-climber and some weight training for a few weeks, then go for a stationary bicycle and a stretch class. If you did that at home, you'd be spending more money on new equipment and videos every few weeks!

One other thing you can do at a health club that you probably can't do at home—*swim*. If you have arthritis or any other joint problem, or if you're extremely heavy and afraid for your knees and your back, having access to a pool can be a real lifesaver. Water aerobics are excellent for anyone with these concerns, and they're fun, too! I was surprised to discover when I tried water aerobics that they use dumbbells—only they're made out of Styrofoam, so the resistance comes from forcing them under the water! Water running is another exercise that's catching on—you wear a flotation belt and run in place in the water. Excellent!

Be aware, though, that while swimming will improve your heart and lungs and up your energy, it's not great for burning fat. Your body seems to know what kind of exercise you're doing, and it will shape itself for that particular stress—and in swimming, a bit of fat is of benefit, both for buoyancy and as insulation. Accordingly, swimming won't slim you down like some other things. Just look at the women who swim the English Channel. Fit? You bet. Skinny? No. But swimming and other water exercises can help you get in good enough shape to do some other things! (Because of the resistance training they incorporate, water aerobics are likely to get you in better shape than just swimming laps.) If there's no health club with a pool near you, try calling some of the local hotels. Often they'll let you pay a monthly fee to use their pool; a friend of my mother's did this for years.

Gyms—The Downside

On the negative side, working out at a gym—unless you live or work right next door—takes more time than working out at home. This is why I'm currently taking the work-out-at-home route. I have taken to "Heavyhand walking"—walking with hand and ankle weights—instead of going to the gym, because I can walk out the door, do my 3.5 mile circuit of my neighborhood, get back home, shower, and change in the time it would take me to get to the gym, change clothes twice, and return home. Add driving time plus changing time, and you're talking at least forty-five minutes—and that doesn't include the workout! In this busy day and age, time is a big issue for a lot of us.

If you're extremely shy about working out in public, a gym can be kind of scary. You might look for a gym that has classes just for people who are overweight; there are some out there. There are also "ladies only" gyms for women who are uncomfortable working out in front of men.

Also, of course, joining a gym costs *money*. For the cost of a month or two at a gym, you could buy a good aerobics-with-weights video and a few dumbbells and get good results at home. Further, your video and weights would then be paid for, but with most gyms, you pay a fee every month.

Getting Fit at Home

How about working out at home? Certainly it's very possible to get into good shape at home, and you don't have to spend a ton of money on fancy equipment to do it. If you have a television and a VCR, your local video rental joint or library audiovisual room is likely to have all the exercise videos you could ever need! Again, I'd recommend that you pick one that includes weights, and invest in a few sizes of dumbbells; they're inexpensive. Rent a video and try it for a few days, then try another, until you find a few you really like. Then you can purchase! An ideal home fitness video library contains aerobics, strength training, and stretching-type videos, all three.

I would like to say here that the very best workout videos I've ever done are put out by a company called *The Firm*. They're just "dance-y" enough to be fun, but not so much so that this klutz can't keep up. They do an excellent job of incorporating weights into the workout, so that you get strength training at the same time you get your aerobic workout, saving you precious time. They're clear and easy to follow—a virtue not to be underestimated. Furthermore, by using heavier or lighter weights, or none at all to start, they can be adapted for just about any level of fitness. *The Firm* videos, in my opinion, are the best of the best. Their "fanny lifter" is a very useful piece of equipment, too, although I improvised for years with various stuff around the house—my kitchen step stool, a cinder block, a very sturdy coffee table.

I purchased Leslie Sansone's *Walk Away the Pounds* videos for my mom for Christmas this year. Since my mom lives in Chicago, being able to walk in place, inside, during the chilly winter—while incorporating some gentle strength training to keep her bones strong—struck me as a *great* idea. I have *never* seen a negative review of these tapes. In particular, people like the fact that there are no dance moves involved. Mom says she's using these tapes and enjoys them. You can find the *Walk Away the Pounds* series at discount stores—I bought them at Target.

Recently I bought the *Zumba* Latin dance aerobics tapes—you may have seen the infomercial for these. Unlike *Walk Away the Pounds,* these are *all* dance. The instructions on these tapes are not as explicit as they should be, and it took me a good week of practice to get the steps on the basic *Zumba* tape down. However, *Zumba* is the most fun I've ever had doing aerobics. Even my husband likes to *Zumba,* and that's really saying something! I've added light wrist weights to increase intensity, strengthen my cardiovascular system even more, and add muscle. If you try this, *start with very light weights.* I started with one-pounders, and I was already in good shape.

I also bought *Pilates for Dummies* when I saw it for a big $6.99 at Kmart. Pilates is tough! However, it strengthens just about all your muscles in twenty minutes. I find this tape clear and easy to follow—if not easy to do!

One other video series, and then I'll stop making unpaid plugs: *Callanetics,* a series of stretching and strengthening exercises, are *superb* for improving posture, flexibility, and bearing. As a massage therapist, I have recommended these tapes many times for people with posture-related pain problems. Improving your posture will make you look slimmer almost overnight. Start with either the original *Callanetics* tape or the beginner tape. Don't underestimate these seemingly low-key exercises; they're a lot tougher than they look!

If you'd like a near-unlimited supply of great exercise videos for very little money, see if your local public television station broadcasts any exercise shows—many do. You can, of course, tape the show if it comes on while you're at work. You could end up with an excellent fitness video library this way, for just the cost of the blank cassettes.

Of course, videos aren't the only way to get in shape at home. There are a million machines on the market, both for aerobic conditioning and strength training. Which machine is best? Once again, the answer is "the one you'll use." Keeping that in mind, there is a real edge to any home exercise machine that lets you vary your workout. The more different things you can do on it, the better. Also, the more muscles get used, the better the workout. A stationary bike uses your legs; a rowing machine uses your legs, your back, your shoulders, your arms, and your stomach muscles. Guess which will get you in better shape, faster? On the other hand, if you like the bike and hate the rowing machine, get the bike!

On Buying Secondhand Equipment

I have this mental picture of you watching those ubiquitous infomercials for exercise equipment, going back and forth on whether or not you should actually shell out just five easy payments of $49.95 for a chance to get in shape in the privacy of your own home.

Hey, I'm one of you. I actually *enjoy* these exercise equipment infomercials, not to mention exercise equipment, and practically every machine I see, I want! However, unless you have a *much* fatter wallet than I, I cannot recommend that you call that 800 number and order the latest Miracle Machine. You know and I know that there are dismayingly good odds that said Miracle Machine will become a high-priced clothes rack—the dreaded Post-Purchase User Neglect syndrome. It's bad enough to kick yourself for not following through with the exercise program. It's far, far worse to kick yourself for paying hundreds of dollars for the privilege.

Does this opinion mean that I don't have any exercise machines, and don't recommend their use? Not on your life! I have a *houseful* of exercise equipment—I own a Total Gym; a "rider" machine; a rowing machine; a ski machine; a mini-trampoline; an aerobic "step"; a few choice exercise videos; and a modest assortment of dumbbells, wrist weights, and ankle weights. And I actually *use* the stuff, though certainly not all of it every day.

But I have learned a very useful economic lesson (learned, I might add, the expensive way): *Five years ago's hot exercise machine is this year's yard sale fodder.* If you just think back to the infomercials of yesteryear, you may remember that at the time, you were simply *dying* for a Health Rider, or a Nordic Track, or a Soloflex, just as today you are convinced that an Ab Swing or a Bun & Thigh Rocker or Tony Little's Gazelle is the answer to your fitness problems.

Guess what? Health Riders and their knock-off cousins are now $10 to $25, used, and widely available. My Cardio Rider cost me $10, and I had a choice at the time of three similar machines in my local area. Nordic Tracks are now so passé that my local Play It Again Sports says they can't even sell them; surely you're going to pay *far* less than the $200 to $600 that folks were paying ten years ago.

Yet all these now-unfashionable machines still work just as well as they ever did. So long as a machine is sturdy, with smooth action, and you find it agreeable enough that you will actually *use* it, your body does not care if you're working out on a Health Rider or a Gazelle. Trust me on this. Yes, some machines may have an edge over others. Certainly the more muscle groups a machine uses, the faster it will burn fat, but overall, the important thing is just to *get* moving and to *keep* moving. And virtually any well-made exercise machine will let you do that.

Which leads me to another point: When you're buying an exercise machine on a budget, there's a temptation to buy a cheap model. But anything that's going to bear your weight and has moving parts had better be well made if you're planning to use it for very long. Good exercise machines have more comfortable seats and smoother action, are sturdier, and are *far* quieter. Really cheap exercise machines are a total waste of money! They're annoying to use and fall apart quickly. I once bought a cheapie stair-stepper—just two pedals with little hydraulic cylinders—thinking I could use it in front of the television. It was *terrible*. The pedals had different degrees of resistance and moved differently. Oh, not *very* differently, but enough to make it uncomfortable to use. Also, the pedals *slammed* down at every step, jarring my whole body and making a loud thunking noise. I used it about twice, and that was it. For that matter, I found one of those

"E-Z Glider" ski machines at a yard sale—very heavily advertised at the same time that NordicTrack was hot; E-Z Glider was the cheapo knockoff—and it was a total piece of junk. I bet no one ever used it more than once.

When you shop for secondhand exercise equipment, suddenly you can afford the good stuff. That crummy little stepper, new, cost me *twice* what my Cardio Rider cost me used. The Cardio Rider is silent, has smooth action, is fun, and uses the majority of muscles in my body—arms, legs, back, and abs, even a little chest. What a bargain! For that matter, I recently saw the infomercial model of the Total Gym—which runs about $1,200 new, and I bought for $700 used, through eBay—advertised in the classifieds for a big $250, nearly as cheap as the model sold at Kmart and Wal-Mart. (There are several features of the expensive model Total Gym that make it considerably more versatile than the cheap model.)

Another plus to buying used exercise equipment is that you can afford to have more than one machine. I have little doubt that one of the reasons this stuff ends up holding clothes or gathering dust is that people get bored with using the same machine, day after day. When you pay a fraction of the original price, you can afford to have a variety of equipment, dramatically reducing the boredom factor. I've used all of my machines within the past year or so. I tend to use one for several weeks to a few months, then switch to another when I get bored. This is also a way to get around the problem of diminishing returns—my trainer buddy, BJ, assures me that after a couple of months, your body adjusts to whatever sort of workout you're doing, and you start to get less and less benefit from it. Owning a modest variety of equipment lets you cross train and progress steadily toward greater fitness.

One final advantage of buying secondhand equipment: If you discover you simply *loathe* a particular machine, you can generally get your money back by selling it to somebody else. You can't do this with new stuff, because once you've used it, it's used stuff, and you're going to get used prices for it. For instance, I discovered, after paying the price for a spiffy new

Nordic Track and using it for a month or two, that I didn't really like the thing much, and furthermore, it was too noisy for my tastes. Do you think I could sell my now-used NordicTrack for the price I paid for it? Not a chance. But would someone else be willing to buy my Cardio Rider from me for the same $10 I paid for it? Sure, not that I'm interested in selling it.

So get in shape the smart way! Harness other people's Post-Purchase User Neglect syndrome. Keep an eye on your local classified ads, browse eBay.com (although packing and shipping some of these things can cost you), check out Play It Again Sports (or any other local used sporting goods stores), go to yard sales. Try out a machine or two, and see what appeals to you. Put together a cool home gym for a very modest amount of money, and your body—and your wallet—will thank you for it!

Here's a list of the stuff I've gotten used, what I paid, and how I like it:

- Mini-trampoline—Tons of fun, and good even for those who are quite out of shape. Originally around $200, I paid $10 at a yard sale. Picked up another one for my mom, at another yard sale, also for $10.
- Dumbbells—Cast iron, ten-pound size. $1 at a yard sale, would cost at least $20–$25 new.
- Dumbbells—The kind with removable plates, complete with plates totaling eighteen pounds each. Free! Found them in the basement of a house I was renting, left behind by the previous tenant. Don't know how much new, but pretty certain they'd cost more than nothing.
- Heavyhands hand weights—for use while walking and during other aerobic exercise. Free, given to me by a friend who wasn't using them. These, sadly, are no longer made, but they were running about $25 at the time. I adore these and would gladly endorse them if they were still being made.
- Ankle weights—Two sets of four pounds each (which is to say, two pounds per ankle per set). Very useful when working out in front of the TV—and they can be strapped to wrists, as well. $1 per pair at a yard sale.

- Aerobic workout step—Includes sturdy, nontip legs that fold flat for storage. I love this, combined with dumbbells, for getting a good workout in front of the TV. $5.99 at Goodwill.

- Exercise videos from *The Firm*—The absolute cream of the video crop, $3–$4 apiece, from a local Blockbuster that was clearing them out of its collection. Videos by *The Firm* are currently running about $15. Be aware that *The Firm* videos on the infomercial are not the only videos from this fine company. There are a bunch; watch for them.

- *Body Flex* breathing exercise videos—$8 apiece at Play It Again Sports. I was very skeptical about breathing exercises and wasn't about to pay "As Seen on TV" prices for these tapes, but I was so impressed with the results that I then paid retail for two other breathing exercise systems, Oxycise! and Life Lift. *Body Flex* is currently on sale at Home Shopping Network for $31.20, plus $5.95 shipping and handling, so $8 a pop was a deal.

- Karen Voight's *Strong and Smooth Moves* video—$1 at a yard sale. And just as well, too; I don't like this tape. Think I can get my buck back when I hold a yard sale of my own?

- Cardio Rider—$10; I found it listed in the local classified ads. When these things were new, they were a couple of hundred bucks a shot. I like this machine a lot, and find it particularly good for getting the blood moving while wasting time in front of the TV. It's absolutely silent, a quality that I greatly admire in exercise equipment; sturdy; stable; and uses the vast majority of the muscles in my body.

- Total Gym—$700, including packing and shipping, for the infomercial model with all the bells and whistles. I bought this off of eBay. Had I bided my time, I could have gotten one cheaper, but I don't feel ripped off having paid as much as I did—which is still several hundred dollars less than it would have cost me new. The Total Gym is a terrific piece of equipment. It can be used to both strengthen and stretch virtually every muscle in the body, it is sturdy and well made, it's fun to use, and it practically saved my life after my car accident, because it let me gently stretch out all my traumatized muscles. The updated infomercial model—as always, advertised by Chuck Norris and Christie Brinkley, is currently running $1,200.

In Praise of Walking

On the other hand, perhaps you'd rather not work out with equipment. How about taking a walk?

Walking is, in many ways, the ultimate exercise. No, it won't get you in the kind of shape that a couple of hours of weight lifting every day will give you, and it doesn't burn fat quite as quickly as running. But walking has so much to recommend it, that I'd like to give it its due right here.

- Walking is the exercise that takes no training. If you're reading this, chances are you already know how to walk!
- Walking takes no expensive equipment; heck, even name-brand walking shoes aren't really necessary. Unless you have foot or knee problems, any shoes that are comfy, have little or no heel, and don't rub will do.
- You're unlikely to injure yourself walking. I learned from massage therapy that running is one of the highest injury sports around; run long enough and you're very likely to hurt your knees or get shin splints or something. But unless you twist an ankle or try to go from couch potato to doing a five-mile hike on rough terrain overnight, chances are slim that walking will do you anything but good.
- You can walk just about anywhere. You don't need to pay for a club membership. You just walk out the front door and go. If you're on break from work, you can walk up the street and back for fifteen minutes. Walk to a local park. Heck, when faced with nothing else, I've walked in big circles around the parking lot at the office building where I was working. Unless you're someplace that is currently iced over (walking on ice is one of the few ways you might get injured), you can find someplace to walk.
- If you live where the weather is severe, or in an iffy

neighborhood, it's good to know that many malls welcome "mall walkers." My mother takes advantage of a mall near her that opens its doors an hour early every day for walkers; no doubt they hope folks will stay and shop. This lets Mom walk in a controlled climate, in safety. Call your local mall and ask if they allow mall walkers—or just go walk. I did this when I was in Dallas for ten days in the summertime and it was about a zillion degrees in the shade. I went to the nearest mall and walked, every day. Even took my hand weights with me! No one said a word.

- Walking is a great way to get a little sunshine. Oh, I know that we're all supposed to be terrified of the sun these days and avoid it like poison, and I do wear my SPF 15 on my face. But I find it hard to believe that we could have evolved in such a close relationship with the sun and have absolutely no use for it or need for it. I know I get depressed and sluggish in the winter when the sun doesn't peek through for days at a time. Getting sunshine cheers me. Furthermore, it helps normalize your body clock—one of the unsung health problems of modern times is living under artificial light all the time. Sunshine during the day helps your brain release melatonin at bedtime, which will help you get to sleep and have a sound night's rest. And there is emerging evidence that lack of sleep may contribute to obesity!

- Walking, of course, is a fine aerobic exercise. It strengthens your cardiovascular system and burns fat at the same time; an excellent thing. Walking also helps get the blood back up from your legs, helping prevent varicose veins, and improves lymphatic circulation, which is excellent for your immune system.

- As I've proven to myself, walking helps alleviate depression. There have actually been scientific studies showing that walking is effective for relieving mild to moderate depression. And it won't make you gain weight like many antidepressants can!

- Walking can be both a wonderful way to get some private time—I find walking alone to be my meditation—or to spend some time with friends or family. In particular, if you have something you need to talk about with a loved one, getting out of the house and taking a walk together can alleviate much of the pressure and make talking much easier. With men, especially, I've found that they're often more comfortable talking this way than when I'm staring right at them. Try it! And, of course, walking with friends can be just plain fun.
- Walking is a very easy way to get into fitness if you've been terribly out of shape. If you haven't even thought about exercise for years, you can take short walks—even ten to fifteen minutes at a time will improve your fitness and will probably be within your capability. Once you're walking comfortably for fifteen minutes at a brisk pace, you can increase your speed, your duration, or both.

So go for a walk!

I like to use hand weights when I walk (these are special dumbbells, made to be comfortable to carry for long periods of time; they have straps that go across the backs of the hands, so there's no need to grip them strongly), and pump my arms hard to increase my "burn." Another benefit of hand weights is that they made me feel far safer back when I used to walk in the city! I think the results of this sort of exercise are *far* greater than those of walking alone, although there is a modestly increased risk of injury, too. If you're interested in maximizing your fitness walking, I highly recommend that you read *The Heavyhands Walking Book,* by Leonard Schwartz. To learn how to do this sort of exercise at home in front of the TV, you might also dig up the original book, *Heavyhands: The Ultimate Exercise,* by the same author. These books are both currently out of print, sad to say, but your public library may have them, and if they don't, they can get them for you through Inter-library Loan, a service which is usually free of charge. I love Heavyhands and would like to see it become more widespread.

How about running? The tendency of your body to shape itself for a particular type of stress is why running seems to be the best sport for slimming down. You lose upper body mass as your body tries to lighten the load it has to carry. But I can tell you after fifteen years of professional massage experience that running has one of the highest injury rates of any sport. If you really *like* running, and have great feet and knees, go for it. Just be sure you have the best possible shoes; cheap running shoes are a luxury you can't afford. But for the general population, I'm not sure the drawbacks of running don't outweigh the benefits.

What else can you do at home? How about pulling the blinds, putting on music, and dancing like a lunatic for half an hour every day? Bet you could even get any little kids who are home to join in, solving the "How do I watch the kids while I work out?" problem. Dancing's a gas! Who cares if you're not a great dancer? Just move around and have fun. You could get a basket for your bicycle and pedal to the convenience store instead of taking the car. You could use a push mower instead of a ride-on job. You could go to the playground with your four-year-old and do every single thing he or she does!

Then there's always good old basic calisthenics—jumping jacks, crunches, leg lifts, all that stuff you did in PE class as a kid. Push-ups, in particular, are terrific; they build your chest, back, and arms all at once. Calisthenics are free, take no equipment, and can be done in your living room while watching television or listening to music. What more do you want?

Another *very* cool exercise to try at home is the mini-trampoline or rebounder. This is a trampoline three feet across and about eight or ten inches high. You can bounce on it, jump on it, jog on it, do jumping jacks, whatever. It's very easy on your joints and a *lot* of fun! Good ones—you don't want a cheap one; who wants a trampoline to give out under them?—are not cheap, about $200. But this is another item often found used. As I mentioned, I got mine for $10 at a yard sale. I really enjoy the thing! I can run and jump on my mini-tramp for half an hour, forty minutes, and I'll get off feeling more energetic than when I started.

If you want to do strength training at home, you can, of course. Buy some dumbbells; they're not very expensive. You'll want more than one size—I have three-pounders, fives, eights, tens, twelves, and eighteens, but you could start with threes, fives, and eights. Then go to your local public library and get a good book on working out with weights. It'll show you how to isolate your different muscles. Remember to work as many different muscles as you can; uneven muscle development can cause postural problems. Ever noticed how some body builders have shoulders that round forward, making them look a little gorilla-like? That comes from working the big, showy muscles of the chest more than the smaller, less flashy muscles in the back. You can actually make quite a lot of progress by lifting weights at home.

Or, if you prefer, you can use resistance bands. Resistance bands are strips or tubes of rubber, some with handles, some without, that you can use to give resistance instead of weights. There are a lot of advantages to resistance bands! First of all, they're inexpensive. Second, with one band you can work out just about every muscle in your body —it can be difficult to do lower-body weight lifting without machines. Third, resistance bands are very light, so you can take them with you when you travel. (As a person who has carried weights in her luggage, I can tell you that this is an advantage not to be underestimated!) Or you can carry a band in your purse, so you can get in a few minutes of exercise on a lunch hour or coffee break. Resistance bands are available at sporting goods stores and some health clubs. Insist on resistance bands that come with a booklet or chart describing and showing the exercises you can do with them.

The Upside and Downside of Working Out at Home
What are the benefits of working out at home? It's cheap, or can be. It requires no travel time, and therefore may be easier to fit into a busy schedule. It allows you to start working out in private, if you're uncomfortable being seen. It can, in some cases, let you include your family in your work outs, which wouldn't hurt them a bit. It lets you use your television time

productively, which for some of us is no small thing. And there's more opportunity to get your exercise outside in good weather, which can be wonderful!

What are the drawbacks? It's very easy to get off track. For most of us, home is the place where we go to relax, to *stop* working; it can be hard to make yourself get off that couch. It's easy to get distracted, too. The phone rings, your spouse wants something, the dog needs to go out, the kids want your attention—it can be easy to get suckered into feeling that all that stuff is more important than your workout, especially if you're iffy about working out in the first place! If you want camaraderie at home, you'll have to make it yourself, by inviting a friend over or getting a family member to join you—and then they can give you an excuse to skip a day by skipping a day themselves! There's only whichever machines you've decided to pay for and give houseroom to; no switching off now and then to cross-train and prevent boredom. And, of course, there's no staff with fitness certification to give you advice and work out a program for you.

Mix It Up

One other thing to keep in mind: BJ, my trainer friend, assures me that after about nine weeks of doing the same exercise routine, it will start to lose its effectiveness. Your body, clever thing that it is, starts to adapt and doesn't think of that exercise as a stress anymore. You not only will stop making progress, you can even start to slip back a little! (This is why aerobics instructors stay up nights devising new routines—it's not just to entertain you, it's to keep you progressing.)

Now, this doesn't mean that you'll regress all the way to where you were before you started, or our ancestors, who walked long distances all the time, would have eventually had no muscles at all! If the only exercise you can stand to do is walk (or bicycle, or whatever), it still beats the heck out of nothing, despite this 9-Week Rule. But the 9-Week Rule does mean that it's a very good idea to change what you're doing every couple of months. Buy a new video, try some new moves with the weights, try a different machine. If you've been walking on a flat course, try one with hills. If you've been walking on hills, try doing sprints of fast walking on a flat course. Throw your body a curve now and then. Okay?

One last thought about exercise: Never underestimate the power of "incidental exercise"—the five to fifteen minutes of activity we can all work in a few times a day. Park at the farthest edge of the parking lot and walk, take the stairs instead of the elevator, get off the bus or the subway a stop or two early. Stop looking for ways to get machines to do your physical work for you. This kind of thing adds up and can make a real difference, and, best of all, it's really easy to work into the busiest day. (About the funniest thing I've ever seen is the people who drive around the parking lot at the health club, looking for the parking space nearest the door!)

If all of this seems a bit much now, wait till you've been on your chosen low-carb program for a week or two. You'll have so much more energy, exercise won't seem quite so impossible. You just might find yourself moving because you *want* to!

CHAPTER TWENTY-FOUR

A Word to the Wise

I GENUINELY FEEL that the advice I have given you in this book is safe and sound for the vast majority of folks. But there are exceptions to every rule, and when you're dealing with health, it's important to be careful. I'd hate for you to be the exception!

Accordingly, here are a few cautions. Please pay close attention, and take me at my word.

First and foremost, please remember that I am *not* a doctor, nor am I a registered dietician. I am a layperson with a longtime interest in nutrition who has rediscovered a time-honored way of losing weight and improving health that has worked *beautifully* for my friends and me. I am *not* qualified to diagnose, prescribe, or treat any ailment, and this book is NOT intended to do so; *it is for your information only.* If you have health problems, you *must* be under a doctor's supervision while shifting over to a low-carbohydrate diet.

This is *especially* true if you have any of the health problems that I talked about being associated with hyperinsulinemia. If you have high blood pressure and are on medication for it, you *must* be supervised. Your blood pressure may well drop so fast on a low-carbohydrate diet that your medication will need adjusting. This is a *good* thing, but we don't want anyone fainting at the grocery store!

If you are diabetic, once again, you may very well need an adjustment in your medication after going low carb. I have one cyberpal with type II diabetes who is medication-free as long as she sticks to her diet. Again, this is a good thing, but you *must be monitored*. Insulin shock is no joke.

As for people with cholesterol and triglyceride problems: Triglycerides tend to drop *very* quickly on a low-carbohydrate diet, and for *most* people cholesterol does, too. But, as I mentioned, there is a minority who will experience a rise in LDL cholesterol, as well as an increase in HDL and a drop in triglycerides, whether from saturated fats or arachidonic acid, no one seems to be quite certain. Most of you will find that you can eat beef and egg yolks, and many other things, and keep your cholesterol low, so don't go assuming that you have to have whites-only omelets. However, you need to be aware of your own blood stats so you can catch it if you're in that minority. Don't fly blind! Get tested, regularly.

Then there are people with kidney damage, like my friend Rob. Most people should have no kidney trouble with this diet. There has been a recent, well-documented, peer-reviewed medical study that shows no difference in kidney function between people who have eaten high-protein diets for years and people who have eaten low-protein, high-carbohydrate vegetarian diets. However, high protein levels are still *very* controversial for people with malfunctioning kidneys, and Rob did *not* eat high protein—he stuck to his minimum protein requirement. If you have kidney problems, you will need to calculate your minimum protein requirement and stay at that level, adding fats to get more calories. Once again, you should certainly be under a doctor's supervision, and be tested *frequently* for kidney function. I would recommend that you try the Carb Controlling or Careful Carb approach, rather than the Basic Low-Carb Diet, if you have *any* kidney trouble at all—and *stay out of ketosis!*

As I mentioned, many people will find their mental health greatly improved by this diet; I've heard it over and over. And if you're fundamentally healthy, psychologically, I see no reason not to try St. John's wort or 5-HTP, in moderation. But if you are being treated for depression or any other mental problem, *do not* attempt to adjust your medication without your doctor's input, or give up treatment in favor of the diet, figuring that it will take care of everything for you. If it doesn't—and mental illness is still very poorly understood—you could pay for it with your happiness, your sanity, your relationships, or even your life. Doesn't mean you can't go low carb; doesn't even mean it won't help your mental state. It just means that you don't know *what* it will do if you have a real chemical imbalance, and you need expert help to adjust that biochemistry.

By the way, don't expect your doctor to be excited about this, or to even be accepting. But remember—there is NO nutrition requirement to get through medical school in this country. It is unlikely that your doctor is aware of the medical research backing up this form of dieting—although I do hear, more and more often, about doctors prescribing a low-carb diet for cholesterol trouble, high blood pressure, or diabetes; it's starting to happen. I would suggest that you tell your doctor you would "like to try it," and that you want him/her to monitor your progress for your own safety. The results will speak for themselves. But if you have any health problems at all, *do not* decide to bypass your doctor and go it alone. "Better safe than sorry" didn't become a cliché for no reason, you know.

Finally, don't make the mistake one girl I know did. She had been on a low-fat, high-carb diet, but she saw my success with low carb. She decided to add fat back into her diet—but kept pigging out on low-fat cookies and chips. She GAINED weight. Bad idea. Low carb only works when it's really low carb. Bottom line: Use your brain, take care of yourself! Good advice no matter what you're doing.

The Rest Is up to You!

I was trying to figure out what to say to you to wind up this book, when fate stepped in. My husband is a member of a fraternal order, and we went to the annual fair at the retirement/nursing home funded by and for members of the order and their families. It was a real down-home event, in a small Midwestern town—people of all ages, lots of crafts for sale, a tractor pull, a parade, many prayers and invocations, several bands, a merry-go-round and camel rides for the kids—and, of course, food.

Bad food. Dangerous food. Barbeque beef made with shreds of meat in a sauce as sugary as pancake syrup, served on white flour buns. Pork tenderloins, breaded and deep-fried, also on white flour buns. Sugar-loaded baked beans. Coleslaw with so much sugar, it was an insult to the cabbage. Lovely ripe red strawberries—sliced and sugared till they were syrupy. Elephant ears—big rounds of fried white flour dough sprinkled with cinnamon sugar. Oceans of soda pop. In fact, there was only one food item I would have been willing to put in my body; the green beans. I didn't bother; I had a glass of iced tea, and just enjoyed the activities. Needless to say, I'd had my eggs for breakfast.

But here's the point of all this: At a conservative estimate, 75 percent of the people there were obese. Just about everybody over forty was not only obese, but looked unwell. Even the kids were overweight; every single one of the girls in the teens club had a double chin—they looked about seventeen years old and they were already on the road to ill health, the misery of obesity, and an early death.

I don't mean to cut these people down. It was a *lovely* crowd, happy and friendly and family-oriented, good and kind and reverent. They were a pleasure to be around. That is why it hurt me, really hurt me, to see so many of them looking *so* unhealthy; to see the children well on their way to a lifetime of health problems. They cheerfully feasted on what they no doubt considered good, down-home cooking, and never once made the connection between the quality of the food they ate, the quality of their health, and the quality of their lives.

How many wives will bury their husbands at all too early an age, struck down by a sudden heart attack? How many women will bury their own sexuality because they hate their own bodies? How many men will be impotent in their prime, from diabetes or just from impaired circulation? How many children will cry themselves to sleep at night from the humiliation heaped on the overweight kids at any school? How many marriages will be ruined by neglect born of simple fatigue? How many family vacations will be canceled because the money is needed for doctor bills? How many deadly drug and alcohol habits will grow from the poisoned soil of sugar addiction? How much simple human misery will result from the thoughtless consumption of "food" that doesn't even merit the title?

Nutrition isn't just about what size jeans you can fit into, although you'll never catch me complaining about having to buy smaller ones. Nutrition is about life, *your* life. You genuinely *are* what you eat, and the quality of your health, your thoughts, your work, your moods, your *life* is not just related to what you eat, it is directly dependent on it.

Life is full of choices; that's what freedom is all about. Choices make life both interesting and often maddeningly difficult. You have the choice before you now to change your life dramatically for the better—not just to lose weight and look better, but to be happier, more energetic, sexier, healthier. To live longer, and *far* better. It's a free choice, completely up to you. All you have to do to get started is *choose*.

But it's not just a choice you can make *now* and be done with it. That would be too easy! It's a choice you'll have to make again and again and again, every meal, every snack, every time you're confronted by the garbage that passes as food all over this grand land of ours. Once you've learned how good it feels to feed your body right, that choice becomes easier and easier, but it's still a choice—a choice between eating what you've become habituated to, and eating real food that will make your body and mind as well as they can be. And should you make a choice one day that you later decide was a mistake, all it takes to get back on track is to make a different choice with your next meal.

I know how hard it is to imagine not eating the food you grew up on. I've been there. Not so long ago, I ate cold cereal for breakfast every morning and pasta for dinner three or four nights a week. But I chose to try a low-carbohydrate diet for just a few weeks, to see how it worked and how I felt—and it changed my life so dramatically for the better, I've been choosing to continue every day, every meal, ever since. I sincerely hope that you can find the extraordinary improvement in your life that a low-carbohydrate diet has brought me and mine.

May all your choices be wise and beneficial and bring you health and happiness.

Internet Resources

ERE, IN NO particular order, are some Web sites that you may find useful and/or interesting. Please keep in mind that although these Web addresses were all current when this book was revised, Web sites come and go, and Web addresses often change. However, a quick search in your favorite search engine under "Low-Carbohydrate Diet" should turn up tons of information.

Hold the Toast!—Okay, I lied about these being in no particular order. Hold the Toast is *my* Web site! Home of Lowcarbezine! —the *free* Internet e-mail newsletter for low-carb dieters, so go subscribe *now*! Plus, there are a few years' worth of back issues in the archives for you to read your way through!
HTTP://WWW.HOLDTHETOAST.COM

The USDA National Nutrient Database for Standard Reference—Put this site on your "favorites" list! A *huge* searchable database of nutritional information on thousands of different foods. It will tell you not only the carbohydrate, protein, fat, and fiber counts, but also pretty much every single nutrient known to humankind. A tremendous boon and one of my favorite examples of our tax dollars at work.
HTTP://WWW.NAL.USDA.GOV/FNIC/CGI-BIN/NUT_SEARCH.PL

PubMed—A public portal to the Medline Database. This is the ultimate resource for the aspiring health sciences geek: A searchable database of more than 12 million medical journal articles, the vast majority of them with abstracts that explain, in brief, how a study was done, and what the results and conclusions were. I've been known to blow away *hours* at this Web site, running one search after another just to see what comes up. Maybe I need to get out more?

HTTP://WWW.PUBMED.COM

HTTP://WWW.NCBI.NIH.GOV/ENTREZ/QUERY.FCGI

The World's Biggest Fad Diet (and Why You Should Probably Avoid It) by Dean Esmay—A terrific article debunking low-fat dieting.

HTTP://WWW.SURVIVEDIABETES.COM/LOWFAT.HTML

Archives of the Low Carb Technical Discussion List— Intelligent, educated people, many of them with degrees in medicine, biochemistry, exercise physiology, or other related disciplines, have been discussing the technical aspects of low-carbohydrate dieting via e-mail for *years* now. Here's a searchable archive of the stuff they've talked about, and a wonderful resource it is, too.

HTTP://MAELSTROM.STJOHNS.EDU/ARCHIVES/LOWCARB.HTML

The Official Atkins Web site—'Nuff said.

HTTP://WWW.ATKINSCENTER.COM

The Soft Science of Dietary Fat—This article, published in the peer-reviewed scientific journal *Science,* won its author, Gary Taubes, the 2001 Science in Society Journalism Award, from the National Association of Science Writers. If you'd like to be astounded by how little scientific support there ever really was for a low-fat/high-carb diet, you *need to read this!*

HTTP://NASW.ORG/MEM-MAINT/AWARDS/01TAUBESARTICLE1.HTML

The same article, with links to interesting commentary:

HTTP://WWW.SECOND-OPINIONS.CO.UK/TAUBES.HTML

Cholesterol and Heart Disease: A Phony Issue—Interesting stuff from Mary Enig, Ph.D., a lipids researcher, stating, among other things, that cholesterol as high as 240 is healthy—and that cholesterol-lowering drugs cause disease. Read this before taking statins!
HTTP://WWW.WESTONAPRICE.ORG/KNOW_YOUR_FATS/FATS_PHONY.HTML

Adiposity 101—A terrific, if long, article about obesity in general, and low-carb diets in specific. This has moved around over the years, so if it's not at this address, do a Web search and you may find it.
HTTP://WWW.OMEN.COM/ADIPOS.HTML

Low Carb Retreat—Many useful resources for the low-carb dieter, including *lots* of low-carb Web links and low-carb chat and discussion groups. Not for those offended by overtly Christian material.
HTTP://WWW.LOWCARBRETREAT.COM/

Low Carb Luxury—A *huge* treasure trove of useful information. Product reviews, book reviews, "beginner's guide," tips and ideas, recipes, an online magazine, a restaurant guide, and much more.
HTTP://WWW.LOWCARBLUXURY.COM/

Atkins Diet & Low Carbohydrate Weight-Loss Support—Especially good source of interesting media articles about low carbing, and the research and the controversy surrounding this way of eating. Also has a link to the text of Banting's *Letter on Corpulence,* the first low-carb diet book! Recipes, success stories, links to low-carb retail Web sites, and more.
HTTP://WWW.LOWCARB.CA/

The Carbohydrate Addict's Official Web site—If the Carb Controlling approach is your diet of choice, this may be your Web site of choice!

HTTP://WWW.CARBOHYDRATEADDICTS.COM/

The alt.support.diet.low-carb Recipe Archives—A huge treasure trove of low-carb recipes, available free!

HTTP://WWW.CAMACDONALD.COM/LC/LOWCARBOHYDRATECOOKING-RECIPES.HTM

Thinner.com—Low-carb online discussion groups, mailing lists, and info about low-carb products.

HTTP://WWW.THINNER.COM/

Low-Carbohydrate Cookbooks

NO DOUBT YOUR standard-issue cookbooks have many recipes that will work for your low-carbohydrate diet, but I think it's helpful to have some low-carb cookbooks, too. A few I'm very fond of include:

500 Low-Carb Recipes, by Dana Carpender, 2002, Fair Winds Press

What, you thought I'd leave out my own cookbook?! No way. It's great. You need it. Go buy it.

The Low-Carb Cookbook, by Fran McCullough, 1997, Hyperion Press

One of the first low-carb cookbooks on the market, and one of the best. Fran is the award-winning author of many cookbooks, and her recipes are wonderful. Her *Living Low-Carb* is worth a read, too. After all, she quotes me!

Dr. Atkins' Quick & Easy New Diet Cookbook, by Robert C. Atkins, M.D., and Veronica Atkins, 1997, Fireside Books

I haven't tried a lot from this, but I've liked what I've tried.

Baking Low Carb, by Diana Lee, 1999, Morris Cookbooks

Bread & Breakfast: Baking Low Carb II, by Diana Lee, 2001, Morris Cookbooks

These books are must-haves for every low-carb kitchen, because they're the only low-carb cookbooks I know devoted solely to baked goods. You'll find recipes for breads, muffins, coffee cakes, cookies, brownies, and more. Absolutely *essential* for the vegetarian low carber! And very useful for all the rest of us. These cookbooks are not available in most bookstores; you can get them through Amazon.com, or you can write down the titles and author and ask your local bookstore to special-order them for you.

Splendid Low Carbing, by Jennifer Eloff, 2000, Eureka Publishing

More Splendid Low Carbing, by Jennier Eloff, 2002, Eureka Publishing

When I flip through Jen's cookbooks, I always find myself thinking, "Why didn't I think of that?" Great recipes and a really nice balance between main dishes, side dishes, desserts, baked goods, etc. *More Splendid Low Carbing* is also notable for having some of the lowest carb counts for the recipes of any low-carb cookbook I've seen, and also for having recipes and menus for doing a fat fast to break a plateau or overcome metabolic resistance. Available through Jen's Web site, http://www.sweety.com.

Bibliography

Books: Starred titles are highly recommended.

Adams, Ruth, & Murray, Frank, *Megavitamin Therapy,* 1980, Larchmont Books

*Allan, Christian B., Ph.D., and Lutz, Wolfgang, MD, *Life Without Bread,* 2000, Keats Publishing

*Atkins, Robert C., M.D., *Dr. Atkins' Health Revolution,* 1989, Bantam Books

*Atkins, Robert C., M.D., *Dr. Atkins' New Diet Revolution,* 1992, M. Evans & Co

*Audette, Ray, *Neanderthin,* 1997, Paleolithic Press

*Davis, Adelle, *Let's Get Well,* 1965, Harcourt, Brace, & World

*Dufty, William, *Sugar Blues,* 1975, Chilton Book Company

Eades, Michael R., M.D., *Thin So Fast,* 1989, Warner Books

*Eades, Michael R., M.D., & Mary Dan, M.D., *Protein Power,* 1996, Bantam

*Fredericks, Carlton, Ph.D., *New Low Blood Sugar and You,* 1985, Perigee Books

*Gittleman, Ann Louise, M.S., C.N.S., *Get the Sugar Out,* 1996, Crown Trade Paperbacks

*Goldberg, Jack, Ph. D., and O'Mara, Karen, D.O., *The GO-Diet,* 1999, GO Corp

Heller, Richard, M.S., Ph. D., & Heller, Rachael, M.A., M.Ph., Ph.D., *Carbohydrate Addicted Kids,* 1997, Harper Collins

Heller, Richard, & Heller, Rachael, *The Carbohydrate Addict's Diet,* 1991, The Penguin Group

*Heller, Richard, & Heller, Rachael, *The Carbohydrate Addict's Lifespan Program,* 1997, The Penguin Group

*Heller, Richard, & Heller, Rachael, *Healthy for Life,* 1995, The Penguin Group

Langer, Stephen E., M.D., and Scheer, James, *Solved: The Riddle of Illness,* 1984, Keats Publishing

MacKarness, Richard, M.D., *Eat Fat and Grow Slim,* 1958, Doubleday

Murray, Michael T., N.D., *The Healing Power of Herbs,* 1995, Prima Publishing

Podell, Richard N., M.D., F.A.C.P., and Proctor, William, *The G-Index Diet,* 1993, Warner Books

Taller, Herman, M.D., *Calories Don't Count,* 1961, Simon and Schuster

Ulene, Dr. Art, *The Nutribase Complete Book of Food Counts,* 1996, Avery Publishing Group

Medical Journal Articles

I want to be honest here, and admit that, in most cases, I read the abstracts of these articles, rather than the full text. Since the abstracts do include the results and conclusions, as well as the methods, of any study, one can learn a lot this way!

Alberts, D.S.; Martinez, M.E.; Roe, D.J.; Guillen-Rodriguez, J.M.; Marshall, J.R.; van Leewen, J.B.; Reid, M.E.; Ritenbaugh, C.; Vargas, P.A.; Bhattacharyya, A.B.; Earnest, D.L.; Sampliner, R.E.

"Lack of effect of a high-fiber cereal supplement on the recurrence of colorectal adenomas." Phoenix Colon Cancer Prevention Physician's Network.

Arizona Cancer Center, Department of Medicine, University of Arizona, Tucson

New England Journal of Medicine, 2000, April 20, 342(16):1156–62

A randomized trial to determine whether dietary supplementation with wheat-bran fiber reduces the rate of recurrence of colorectal adenomas. One thousand four hundred twenty-nine men and women between 40 and 80 years of age, with a recent history of colorectal adenomas, were given either high amounts (13.5 grams per day) or low amounts (2 grams per day) of wheat-bran fiber. The presence or absence of new adenomas was then noted during follow-up colonoscopy. Both subjects and physicians were unaware of which group was getting which quantity of fiber. Median time to follow-up colonoscopy was 34 months in the high-fiber group and 36 months in the low-fiber group. When all follow-up colonoscopies were completed, at least one adenoma had been found in 338 of the subjects in the high-fiber group, and in 299 of the subjects in the low-fiber group. It was concluded that a dietary supplement of wheat-bran fiber does not protect against recurrence of colorectal adenoma.

Augustin, L.S.; Dal Maso, L.; La Vecchia, C.; Parpinel, M.;
Negri, E.; Vaccarella, S.; Kendall, C.W.; Jenkins, D.J.;
Franseschi, S.

"Dietary glycemic index and glycemic load, and breast cancer
  risk: a case-controlled study."

Servizio di Epidemilogia, Centro Di Riferimento Oncologico,
Instituto Nazionale Tumori, Aviano, Italy

Annals of Oncology, 2001, November, 12(11):1533–8

Researchers studied 2,569 women with confirmed breast cancer,
with 2,588 breast cancer–free women as controls. Average daily
glycemic index and glycemic load were calculated from a 78-
item food frequency questionnaire. Direct associations with
breast cancer risk emerged for glycemic index and glycemic load.
High glycemic index foods, such as white bread, increased the
risk of breast cancer, while the intake of pasta, a medium
glycemic index food, seemed to have no influence. Findings were
consistent regardless of menopausal status, alcohol intake, or
physical activity. The hypothesis that there is a direct association
between glycemic index or glycemic load and breast cancer risk,
and therefore a possible role of hyperinsulinemia/insulin resistance in breast cancer development was supported.

Augustin, L.S.; Polesel, J.; Bosetti, C.; Kendall, C.W.; La
Vecchia, C.; Parpinel, M.; Conti, E.; Montella, M.;
Franscheschi, S.; Jenkins, D.J.; Dal Maso, L.

"Dietary glycemic index, glycemic load and ovarian cancer
  risk: a case controlled study in Italy."

Servizio di Epidemilogia, Centro Di Riferimento Oncologico,
Instituto Nazionale Tumori, Aviano, Italy

Annals of Oncology, 2003, January, 14(1):78–84

Because dietary carbohydrates vary in their ability to raise blood
glucose and insulin levels, which, in turn, influences levels of sex
hormones and insulin-like growth factors, the researchers analyzed the effect of type and amount of carbohydrates on ovarian
cancer risk, using both glycemic index and glycemic load meas-
urements. One thousand thirty-one women with confirmed
ovarian cancer were compared with 2,411 women who did not

have ovarian cancer. Average daily glycemic index and glycemic load were calculated from a food frequency questionnaire. Ovarian cancer was directly associated with glycemic index and glycemic load. The association was observed in both pre- and postmenopausal women. The researchers conclude that hyperinsulinemia and/or insulin resistance may play a role in ovarian cancer development.

Axen, K.V.; Li, X.; Fung, K.; Sclafani, A.
"The VMH-dietary obese rat: a new model of non-insulin dependent diabetes mellitus."
(R) *American Journal of Physiology*, 1994, 266:R921–R928.
Rats given a high-fat, high-sucrose diet showed fasting hyperin-sulinism and hypertriglyceridemia within 3 weeks. Fasting hyperglycemia observed in the majority in 7 consecutive experiments. Impaired glucose tolerance was shown despite high prevailing insulin levels. Loss of insulin secretory response to glucose by week 5. Islet cells failed to suppress insulin release normally.

Beck, S.A.; Tisdale, M.J.
"Effect of insulin on weight loss and tumour growth in a cachexia model."
Pharmaceutical Sciences Institute, Aston University, Birmingham, UK
Br. J. Cancer, 1989, May, 59:5, 677–81
Showed that a ketogenic diet was superior to insulin administration for preventing cachexia (wasting) in cancer, and that the ketogenic diet had the added benefit of reducing cancer growth.

Blum, M.; Averbuch, M.; Wolman, Y.; Aviram, A.

"Protein intake and kidney function in humans: its effect on 'normal aging.'"

Department of Nephrology, Rokach Hospital, Tel Aviv, Israel

Archives of Internal Medicine, 1989, January, 149(1):211–2

Study comparing kidney function in healthy people following a "normal" unrestricted protein diet to that in vegetarians eating a long-term low-protein diet. Kidney function was similar, and kidneys were found to be aging at the same rate.

Caprio, S.; Bronson, M.; Sherwin R.S.; Rife, F.; Tamborlane, W.V.

"Co-existance of severe insulin resistance and hyperinsulinemia in pre-adolescent obese children."

Department Pediatrics, Yale University Medical School

Diabetologia, 1996, December, 39:12, 1489–97

Chantre, P.; Lairon, D.

"Recent findings of green tea extract AR25 (Exolise) and its activity for the treatment of obesity."

Laboratoires Arkopharma, Carros, France

Phytomedicine, 2002, January, 9(1):3–8

Green tea extract showed an ability to inhibit fat-digesting enzymes and to stimulate thermogenesis. In a 3-month open study of moderately obese patients, body weight was decreased by 4.6% and waist circumference by 4.48%

Chauhan, A.; Foote, J.; Petch, M.C.; Schofield, P.M.

"Hyperinsulinemia, coronary artery disease, and syndrome X."

Journal of the American College of Cardiology, 1994, 23:364–8

Insulin responses to oral glucose compared in 17 patients with coronary artery disease, 17 with chest pain, positive exercise test finding, normal coronary arteries, and impaired coronary flow reserve (syndrome X), and 17 healthy volunteers. Subjects were matched for age, gender, and weight. Higher insulin levels were found in the CAD and X groups. No significant difference was found between the two groups.

Cordain, L.; Eaton, S.B.; Miller, J.B.; Mann, N.; Holt, S.H.; Speth, J.D.

"Plant-animal subsistence ratios and macronutrient energy estimations in worldwide hunter-gatherer diets."

Department of Health and Exercise Science, Colorado State University, Fort Collins, Colorado

American Journal of Clinical Nutrition, 2000, March, 71(3):682–92

Because hunter-gatherer diets are believed to represent a reference standard for human nutrition, and a model for defense against "diseases of affluence," this study attempts to determine what, exactly, those diets may have consisted of. Looks at the plant-to-animal economic subsistence patterns of hunter-gatherers, the differences in body fat percentages of prey animals, and how this would alter protein intakes and influence the selection of other foods. Analysis shows that whenever and wherever ecologically possible, hunter-gatherers consumed between 45% and 65% of their calories from animal food. Seventy-three percent of worldwide hunter-gatherer societies derive 56%–65% of their subsistence from animal foods; only 14% derive more than 50% of their subsistence from gathered plant foods. "This high reliance on animal-based foods coupled with the relatively low carbohydrate content of wild plant foods produces universally characteristic macronutrient consumption ratios in which protein is elevated at the expense of carbohydrates."

Cordain, L.; Eaton, S.B.; Miller, J.B.; Mann, N.; Hill, K.

"The paradoxical nature of hunter-gatherer diets: meat-based, yet non-atherogenic."

Department of Health and Exercise Science, Colorado State University, Fort Collins, Colorado

European Journal of Clinical Nutrition, 2002, March, 56 Suppl 1S42–52

Researchers analyzed 13 quantitative dietary studies of hunter-gatherers and demonstrated that the dominant energy source (65% of calories) was provided by animal food, with gathered plant food supplying the remainder of calories. This, combined with other evidence, including studies of Paleolithic hominid collagen tissue, enzyme levels, gut size, and foraging data, points toward a long history of meat-based diets in humans. It is seen as paradoxical that hunter-gatherers, who consume a majority of calories from animal foods, are relatively free of the signs and symptoms of cardiovascular disease. The high-protein and low-carbohydrate levels of this diet are referred to as "hypolipidemic." It is speculated that the differences in the fatty acid profiles of game over modern domesticated meat might also be a factor, along with high intakes of antioxidants, fiber, vitamins, and phytochemicals, a low salt intake, and a high-exercise/low-stress lifestyle.

Dulloo, A.G.; Seydoux, J.; Girardier, L.; Chantre, P.; Vandermander, J.

"Green tea and thermogenesis: interactions between catechin-polyphenols, caffeine and sympathetic activity."

Institute of Physiology, University of Fribourg, Fribourg, Switzerland

International Journal of Obesity Related Metabolic Disorders, 2000, February, 24(2):252–8

Study to determine if the thermogenic effects of green tea can be attributed solely to its caffeine content. Green tea extract was determined to have a greater thermogenic effect than could be attributed to caffeine alone. It is suggested that these extra thermogenic properties could reside in an interaction between catechin-polyphenols and caffeine, plus sympathetically released noradrenalin. It is suggested that this could be of value in assisting the management of obesity.

Feskens, E.J.; Loeber, J.C.; Kronhout, D.

"Diet and physical activity as determinants of hyperinsulinemia: the Zutphen elderly study."

American Journal of Epidemiology, 1994, August 15, 140(4):350–60

Insulin levels were shown to inversely associate with fiber and polyunsaturated fatty acid intake.

Franceschi, S.; Dal Maso, L.; Augustin, L; Negri, E.; Parpinel, M.; Boyle, P.; Jenkins, D.J.; La Vecchia, C.

"Dietary glycemic load and colorectal cancer risk."

Servizio di Epidemilogia, Centro Di Riferimento Oncologico, Instituto Nazionale Tumori, Aviano, Italy

Annals of Oncology, 2001, February, 12(2):172–8

Stating that insulin and insulinlike growth factors can stimulate proliferation of colorectal cells, and that high intake of refined carbohydrates and markers of insulin resistance are associated with an increased risk of colon cancer, the researchers determined whether glycemic index and glycemic load were associated with colorectal cancer risk. One thousand one hundred twenty-five men and 828 women with confirmed colon or rectal cancer were studied, with 2,073 men and 2,081 women who did not have colorectal cancer as controls. Daily glycemic index and glycemic load, and fiber intake, were calculated from a food frequency questionnaire. Direct associations with colorectal cancer emerged for glycemic index and glycemic load. Overweight and a low intake of fiber from fruits and vegetables appeared to amplify this association. Researchers conclude that refined carbohydrates play a detrimental role in the development of colon cancer.

Franceschi, S.; Favero, A.; Decorli, A.; Negri, E.; La Vecchia, C.; Ferraroni, M.; Russo, A.; Salvini, S.; Amadori, D.; Conti, E.; et al.

"Intake of macronutrients and risk of breast cancer."

Lancet, 1996, May 18, 347(9012):1351–6

A diet high in fat, especially monounsaturated fat, was shown to correlate with a reduced risk of breast cancer. A diet high in carbohydrates, especially starches, was shown to correlate with an increased risk of breast cancer.

Fuchs, C.S.; Giovannuci E.L.; Colditz, G.A.; Hunter, D.J.; Stampfer, M.J.; Rosner, B.; Speizer, F.E.; Willett, W.C.

"Dietary fiber and the risk of colorectal cancer and adenoma in women."

Department of Medicine, Brigham and Women's Hospital and Harvard Medical School, Boston, Massachusetts

New England Journal of Medicine, 1999, January 21, 340(3):169–76

This study was designed to confirm or disprove the idea that a high intake of dietary fiber reduces the risk of colorectal cancer and adenoma. Eighty-eight thousand seven hundred fifty-seven women, 34–59 years old, with no history of cancer, inflammatory bowel disease, or familial polyposis, completed a dietary questionnaire in 1980. During a 16-year follow-up period, 787 cases of colorectal cancer were documented in this group. Further, 27,530 of the women underwent endoscopy, and 1,012 patients with adenomas of the distal colon and rectum were found among them. After adjusting for age, established risk factors, and total energy (calorie) intake, no association between the intake of dietary fiber and the risk of colorectal cancer was found. No protective effect of dietary fiber was observed.

Garg, A.; Bantle, J.P.; Henry, R.R.; Coulston, A.M.; Griver, K.A.; Roatz, S.K.

"Effects of varying carbohydrate content of diet in patients w/non-insulin-dependant diabetis mellitus."

Journal of the American Medical Association, May 11, 271(8):1421–8

High-carbohydrate diet was shown to increase fasting plasma triglycerides and VLDL by 24% and 23% respectively, as contrasted with a diet high in monounsaturated fatty acids, and was also shown to increase insulin levels by 10%. In NIDDM patients, high-carbohydrate diets compared with high MUFA diets caused persistant deterioration of glycemic control and accentuation of hyperinsulinemia, increased triglycerides, and VLDL.

Garg, A.; Grundy, S.M.

"High carbohydrate, low fat diet?"

Hosp. Proct. Off. Ed., 1992, February, 27 Suppl. 1:11–14, discussion on 14–16

Researchers found that triglyceride levels rise in response to increased carbohydrate intake in normal children. Moreover, carbohydrate raises blood glucose levels and insulin requirements

Giovannucci, E.

"Insulin and colon cancer."

Channing Laboratory, Department of Medicine, Harvard Medical School, Boston, Massachusetts

Cancer Causes and Control, 1995, March, 6(2):164–79

Stating that the fat and fiber hypothesis of colon cancer etiology does not explain emerging findings, this researcher looks at the hypothesis that hyperinsulinemia promotes colon cancer. Specifically, he states that the factors that are associated with colon cancer risk are similar to those that are associated with elevated insulin levels: central (abdominal) obesity, physical inactivity, a diet high in refined carbohydrates and low in water-soluble fiber causing a rapid absorption of glucose, leading to postprandial hyperinsulinemia.

Gould, K.L.; Casscells, S.W.; Buja, L.M.; Goff, D.C.

"Non-invasive management of coronary artery disease: report of a meeting at the University of Texas Medical School at Houston."

Department of Internal Medicine, University of Texas Medical School, Houston

The Lancet, 1995, September 16, 346(8977):750–3, Related Articles, Links

Study concerned one 68-year-old male with high cholesterol and a family history of heart disease. Patient was prescribed a low-fat, high-carbohydrate diet and medication. At the end of 1 year, testing was done, and cholesterol had increased. Medication was adjusted, and dietary fat was cut back to 10% of calories. At next testing, mild improvement was noted.

Hunter, D.J.; Speigelman, D.; Adami, H.O.; Beeson, L.; van den Brandt, P.A.; Folsom, A.R. Fraser, G.E.; Goldbohm, R.A.; Graham, S.; Howe, G.R.; et al.

"Cohort studies of fat intake and the risk of breast cancer—a pooled analysis."

Department of Epidemiology, Harvard School of Public Health, Boston, Massachusetts

New England Journal of Medicine, 1996, February 8, 334(6):356–61

Stating that most cohort studies do not confirm an association between fat intake and breast cancer, but have been criticized for involving small numbers of cases, for homogenous fat intake and for measurement errors, the authors identified seven studies in 4 countries that fit specific criteria, and analyzed the data in a standardized manner. Information about 4,980 cases of breast cancer from studies including 337,819 women was available. When the women with the highest fat intake were compared to the women with the lowest fat intake, the risk of cancer was very nearly identical. The authors found no evidence of a positive association between total dietary fat intake and the risk of breast cancer. There was no reduction in risk even among women whose fat intake was less than 20% of calories. It was concluded that lowering total fat intake is unlikely to reduce breast cancer risk substantially.

Jeppesen, J.; Schaaf, P.; Jones, C.; Zhou, M.Y.; Chen, Y.D.; Reaven, G.M.

"Effects of low-fat, high-carbohydrate diets on risk factors for ischemic heart disease in postmenopausal women."

Department of Medicine, Stanford University School of Medicine

American Journal of Clinical Nutrition, 1997, April, 65(4):1027–33

Concluded that recommending a low-fat, high-carbohydrate diet for prevention of heart disease in postmenopausal women was questionable, owing to deleterious effects on blood lipid levels.

Katan, Martijn B.

"Effect of low-fat diets on plasma high-density lipoprotein concentrations."

Department of Human Nutrition, Wageningen Agricultural University, Wageningen, Netherlands

The American Journal of Clinical Nutrition, 1998, March, 67:3

Found that low-fat, high-carbohydrate diets lead to lower HDL levels, and thus higher theoretical risk of heart disease. Weight loss on low-fat diets was found to be insufficient to offset this risk.

Ludwig, D.S.; Majzoub, J.A.; Al-Zahrani, A.; Dallal G.E.; Blanco, I.; Roberts, S.B.

"High glycemic index foods, overeating, and obesity."

Division of Endocrinology, Department of Medicine, Children's Hospital, Boston, 300 Longwood Ave, Boston, Massachusetts

Pediatrics, 1999, March, 103(3):E26

Study looked at the effects of meals with the same calorie count, but varying glycemic indices, on subsequent hunger. Twelve obese teenaged boys were participants and were fed identical test meals for breakfast and lunch, with the same caloric content but differing glycemic indices. Food intake for the rest of the day was monitored. Caloric intake was 53% greater after the high-GI meal than after the medium-GI meal, and 81% greater than after the low-GI meal. The high-GI meal led to higher serum insulin levels and lower plasma glucagon levels. It was concluded that the rapid absorption of glucose after high-GI meals induces a sequence of hormonal and metabolic changes that promote excessive food intake in obese subjects.

Martinez, F.J.; Rizza, R.A.; Romero, J.C.

"High-Fructose feeding elicits insulin resistance, hyperinsulinism, and hypertension in normal mongrel dogs."

Hypertension, 1994, April, 23(4):456–63

Researchers concluded that chronic high-fructose feeding elicits hypertriglyceridemia, insulin resistance, hyperinsulinemia, hypertension, and transient sodium retention in dogs.

Nebeling, L.C.; Lerner, E.

"Effects of a ketogenic diet on tumor metabolism and nutritional status in pediatric oncology patients: two case reports."

Journal of the American College of Nutrition, 1995, April, 14:2, 202–8

Two pediatric cancer patients were given a ketogenic diet high in medium-chain triglycerides. A 21.8% decrease in glucose uptake by the tumor was shown in both patients. One patient, showing a marked improvement in mood and learning on the ketogenic diet, remained on the diet for 12 months, during which time the cancer did not progress.

Nebeling, L.C.; Lerner, E.

"Implementing a ketogenic diet based on medium-chain triglyceride oil in pediatric patients with cancer."

Journal of the American Dietetic Association, 1995, June, 95:6, 693–7

A ketogenic diet high in medium-chain triglycerides was fed to pediatric cancer patients to maintain weight while lowering glucose available for tumor metabolism.

Nobels, F.; van Gaal, L.; de Leeuw, I.

"Weight reduction with a high protein, low carbohydrate, calorie-restricted diet: effects on blood pressure, glucose, and insulin levels."

Netherlands Journal of Medicine, 1989. December, 35:5–6, 295–302

Showed that high blood pressure was tied to blood glucose levels, and that a high-protein, low-carbohydrate weight loss diet successfully lowers blood pressure and helps to improve glucose metabolism.

Reaven, G.M.

"Abnormalities of carbohydrate and lipoprotein metabolism in patients with hypertension; relationship to obesity."

Stanford University Medical School

Annals of Epidemiology, 1991, May, 1:4, 304–11

Simonson, D.C.

"Hyperinsulinemia and its sequelae."

Department of Internal Medicine, Joslin Diabetes Center, New England Deaconess Hospital, Boston, Massachusetts

Horm. Metab. Res. Suppl., 1990;22:17-25. Review

Skov, A.R.; Toubro, S.; Bulow, J.; Krabbe, K.; Parving, H.H.; Astrup, A.

"Changes in renal function during weight loss induced by high vs. low-protein diets in overweight subjects."

Research Department of Human Nutrition, The Royal Veterinary and Agricultural University, Copenhagen, Denmark.

International Journal of Obesity Related Metabolic Disorders, 1999, November, 23(11):1170–7

Six-month study of 65 healthy overweight and obese subjects, given diets where either 25% or 12% of calories came from protein; the fat fraction remained constant at 30%. Adaptive changes in kidney size and function were observed, without indications of adverse effects.

Sowers, J.R.; Standley, P.R.; Ram J.L.; Zemel, M.B.; Resnick, L.M.

"Insulin resistance, carbohydrate metabolism, and hypertension."

Division of Endocrinology, Wayne State University, Michigan

American Journal of Hypertension, 1991, July, 4:7 Pt. 2, 4665–4725

Tisdale, M.J.; Brennan, R.A.

"A comparison of long-chain triglycerides and medium-chain triglycerides on weight loss and tumours in a cachexia model."

Pharmaceutical Sciences Institute, Aston University, Birmingham, United Kingdom

British Journal of Cancer, 1988, November, 58:5, 580–3

In animal studies, a ketogenic diet high in medium-chain triglycerides reduced wasting and caused a "marked reduction in tumour size."

Willett, W.C.; Stampfer, M.J.; Colditz, G.A.; Rosner, B.A.; Hennekens, C.H.; Speizer, F.E.

"Dietary fat and the risk of breast cancer."

New England Journal of Medicine, 1987, January 1, 316(1):22–8

In 1980, 89,538 registered nurses between 34 and 59 years of age, with no history of cancer, completed a dietary questionnaire designed to measure individual consumption of total fat, saturated fat, linoleic acid, and cholesterol, as well as other nutrients. A subsample of 173 participants was studied in greater detail, and it was found that those with the highest fat intake were deriving a mean of 44% of their calories from fat, as compared with 32% in the lowest quintile (fifth). During 4 years of follow up, 601 cases of breast cancer were found among the 89,538 participants. The women in the quintile (fifth) with the highest fat intake were found to have a lower risk of cancer than the women in the quintile (fifth) with the lowest fat intake. The results were similar for pre- and postmenopausal women.

Williams, P.T.; Krauss, R.M.; Stefanick M.L.; Vranizan K.M.; Wood P.D. *Metabolism*, 1994, May; 43(5):655-63

"Effects of low-fat diet, calorie restriction and running on lipoprotein subfraction concentrations in moderately overweight men."

Researchers studied the effect of exercise (primarily running), calorie restriction, and low-fat/high-carbohydrate diet on changes in lipoprotein subfractions in moderately overweight men. After 1 year, complete data were obtained from both those simply dieting and those combining dieting with running. Both groups reduced weight. No significant changes were found in lipoprotein mass and HDL in dieters who did not run.

Yamasaki, R.; Miyoshi, T.; Imaki, M.; Nakamura, T.
"Evaluation of the effects of various factors on the serum triglyceride level in young adults."
Tokushima Journal of Experimental Medicine, 1994, June, 41(1–2):17–30
The researchers carried out surveys and laboratory studies on relationships of nutritional intake, physical activity, cigarette smoking, and alcohol consumption of young adults with serum triglyceride levels. Nutritional survey indicated significant correlation between the serum triglyceride levels and carbohydrate intake. Exercise caused a slight but not significant decrease.

Popular Press Articles

Brody, Jane E. "A new study sees no link between a low-fat diet and breast cancer. Is this the final word? Not likely."
New York Times, February 14, 1996.

Challem, Jack, "Paleolithic nutrition: Your future is in your dietary past." *Nutrition Science News,* April 1997.

La Voie, Angela. "Low-fat diets can have undesired effects."
Medical Tribune News Service, March 21, 1997.

"Link between fatty diet, breast cancer disputed."
The Detroit News, February 8, 1996.

"Low-fat diet may not affect women's breast cancer risk."
USA Today, April 27, 1998.

Meyer, Tara. "Diabetes reaches record levels in the U.S."
Associated Press, May 1, 1998.

News from the Rockefeller University. "Low fat, high sugar diets prompt production of saturated fats." January 23, 1998.

Reuters. "Study links low cholesterol to violent death." March 14, 1998.

Richards, Mike. "'First Farmers' with no taste for grain." *British Archaeology,* March 1996, no.12. Bone analysis suggests Neolithic people preferred meat.

Ritter, Malcolm. "People are talking—Health: Diabetes becomes more prevalent as Americans age, don't exercise." *The Detroit News,* November 3, 1995.

"Study shows danger of fat in margarine." *The Herald-Times,* Bloomington, IN, November 20, 1997.